Freedom From Fat
The Unbridled Truth about Weight Gain
and
How to Take Off Your Weight for Life

By Chris Tomshack, D.C.
Patrick K. Porter, Ph.D.
And the Doctors at
HealthSource® Chiropractic

Foreword By
Dr. Kevin Huffman, DO

Other Books, Audios & Events
By HealthSource Chiropractic
www.healthsourcechiro.com

Cover Art & Graphics : Jason Rina (isuktagum10@gmail.com)

Disclaimer: This book is designed to provide information in regard to the subject matter covered. It is sold with the understanding that the publisher and author are not engaged in rendering psychological advice. The processes in this book are non-diagnostic and non-psychological. If psychological or other expert assistance is required, the services of a licensed professional should be sought. The purpose of this book is to educate and entertain. The publisher, author, or any dealer or distributor shall not be liable to the purchaser or any other person or entity with respect to any liability, loss, or damage caused or alleged to be caused directly or indirectly by this book. If you do not wish to be bound by the above, you may return this book for a full refund.

First Edition: January 2010

Published by PorterVision Publishing. Copyright 2009 by Chris Tomshack, DC and Patrick K. Porter, Ph.D. All rights reserved. No part of this publication may be reproduced or transmitted in any form or by any means, electronic or mechanical, including photocopy, recording or any information storage system now known or to be invented without permission in writing from HealthSource Chiropractic except by a reviewer who wishes to quote brief passages in connection with a review written for inclusion in a magazine, newspaper, video, or broadcast. Violation is a federal crime, punishable by fine and/or imprisonment. Title 17, U.S.C. Section 104.

ISBN: 978-0-615-34623-6
Printed in the United States of America
10 9 8 7 6 5 4 3 2

Table of Contents

Dedication	*11*
Acknowledgement	*11*
Foreword - Kevin Huffman, DO	*13*
Introduction	
by Chris Tomshack, DC	*15*

Chapter One: The Acid/Base Balance
by Richard Kearns, DC — **21**

The College Discovery That Changed My Life	*22*
How To Check Your pH	*23*
How Do Symptoms Develop From Too Much Acid?	*24*
Do you notice anything about the base-yielding foods compared to the acid-forming foods?	*27*
What Roll Does Stress Play?	*29*
Tips For Keeping Your pH At A Optimal Level	*31*

Chapter Two: Oxygenating the Body – The Lymphatic System
by Chad Young, DC — **33**

What is the Lymphatic System and Why is it Important?	*34*
Lymphedema and Our Weight	*35*
Oxygen--the Fountain of Youth?	*36*
Helping the Lymphatic System Perform at its Peak	*37*
Rebounding	*39*

Chapter Three: Detoxifying the Body and Weight Loss
by Joseph Hayes, DC — **43**

Preparing Your Body Is Key To Weight Loss	*44*
The Natural Side Benefit Is Weight Loss	*44*
My Detox Journey	*45*
What roll does the liver play?	*46*
Working with the experts	*47*
Tips to Detoxifying	*47*
Watch out for the Road Blocks	*49*
The Importance of the Four R's	*48*
Increasing Water Is The First Step	*50*
Success Is Up To You!	*51*

CHAPTER FOUR: FEEDING THE BODY -- BODY CHEMISTRY
BY AMANDA BORRE, DC — 53

- What is Lactose? — 55
- What is a Complex Carbohydrate? — 56
- What does Amylase Do? — 56
- What is the Process of Glycolyis? — 57
- What's So Important About Insulin? — 58
- How Important Is Quantity? — 59
- How do we even know about the existence of sugar? — 59
- What's the Good Part? — 60
- What about Bread? — 61
- Do You Have A Plan? — 62

CHAPTER FIVE: DISPELLING THE MYTHS – PROTEIN
BY FRANK DACHTLER, DC — 65

- What is Protein? — 67
- Does too much protein cause Kidney issues? — 68
- Who is likely to have protein deficiency? — 70
- Are all proteins the same? — 70
- What are incomplete proteins? — 71
- Is it really possible to eat more and weigh less? — 72
- What happens on a high protein diet? — 73

CHAPTER SIX: SUGAR AWARENESS
BY BRANDON PETTKE, DC — 75

- Some Amazing Sugar Stats! — 76
- Types of Sugars — 77
- The Most Consumed "Sugar"... It's Everywhere! — 77
- How HFCS Is Made? — 78
- "Health Foods" With HFCS — 79
- If HFCS Is So Bad, Then Why Is It Everywhere? — 80
- Glycemic Index: What The Heck Is This? — 81
- Insulin: Too Much Of It, For Too Long Will Get You Fat & Keep You Fat — 82
- Insulin Resistance: What You Will Get If You Do The Previous High Glycemic Scenario Too Long — 86
- Study on Artificial Sweeteners — 88
- Findings From the Study — 88

So What Should I Eat Then!?	92
Here is a short list/guideline for you (high GI and GL foods):	93
What Should I Take From This Chapter?	94

CHAPTER SEVEN: IMPORTANCE OF FIBER IN WEIGHT LOSS AND HEALTH
BY JESSI REZAC, MS — 95

What is Fiber?	96
Fiber and Weight Loss	97
My Secret Belly Slimming Breakfast	98
How Can I Get More Fiber in MY Diet?	99

CHAPTER EIGHT: THE ROLL OF ENZYMES IN HEALTH AND WEIGHT LOSS
BY MASON ORTH, DC — 103

An Introduction to Digestive Health	105
Macronutrients and micronutrients -- What are they and how do they impact your health?	105
Digestion -- The Journey to Health	107
Proper Energy?	108
Enzymes -- the Key to Proper Digestion	109
Enzyme Depletion	110
Symptoms of Enzyme Depletion	112
How can you treat low Enzyme Levels?	113
Enzymes and Your Weight Loss Goals	113

CHAPTER NINE: THE IMMUNE SYSTEM AND WEIGHT LOSS
BY MICHAEL J. PORTER, BS — 115

What Is Your Immune Response?	116
What is Agglutination?	117
Do You Have Food Sensitivity?	119
Could Reactive Foods Be The Cause Of Weight Gain?	122
What Is Exercising Roll with Food Sensitivity?	125
Is False Fat To Blame?	126
How To Test For Trigger Foods?	128
What Does The Research Say?	130
What Can You Do?	132
What's Your Next Step?	134

CHAPTER TEN: CHANGING YOUR BELIEFS ABOUT WEIGHT LOSS
BY PATRICK K. PORTER, PH.D. **137**

What is Visualization? 139
Why Creative Visualization? 142
What is the Relaxation Response? 143
Why use Creative Visualization
and Guided Relaxation Together? 144
What's the right-brain got to do with it? 144
What's the Left-brain Got to Do With It? 145
How Will Behavioral Repatterning Help You
Reduce Stress and Lose Weight? 146
How Can Behavioral Repatterning Help You
Unleash Your Inner Artist? 147
How Can You Use Logic As a Lever? 148
What Can Your Left-Brain Do for You? 149
What Can Your Right-brain Do for You? 151
Seventeen Characteristics of a Right-brain Thinker 152
Thought Experiment: How Are You Wired? 153
What are the Benefits of Whole-Brain Thinking? 156
Six Major facts About Whole-Brain Thinking 157
What is this Magic Elixir that Can
Transform Your Life and the World? 157

CHAPTER ELEVEN: FATS YOUR BODY NEEDS AND WHY – ESSENTIAL FATTY ACIDS
BY CHRIS TOMSHACK, DC **159**

What are Essential Fats? 161
Why Worry About HDL and LDL? 161
Why Do Our Bodies Need "Good Fat"? 162
What is ALA and How Can You Get It? 163
Can Eating the Right Fat Save Your Heart? 163
What Does the Research Say You Should Do? 164
What's the Right Amount For You? 166
Adding Essential Fatty Acids to Your Diet. 167
A Plan For Those That Don't Like Fish 168
Your Next Step 169

CHAPTER TWELVE: REVERSING THE AGING PROCESS AND WEIGHT LOSS
BY JEREMY BUSCH, DC — **168**

"You Are What You Eat"... Yeah!	174
Inflammation and Prostaglandins:	176
Fatty Acid Imbalance: Omega 6 vs. Omega 3	177
O6AA: Omega 6 Addiction Anonymous!	178
Set Free with Omega 3:	179
115 Pound Weight Loss in 7 months:	183
Anti-inflammatory Recipes:	184
Conclusion:	190

CHAPTER THIRTEEN: METABOLISM -- NATURAL NUTRIENTS VS. STIMULANTS
BY ANDY NELSON, DC — **195**

A Novel Discovery with an Unexpected Twist	196
It Just Gets Better	197
Leptinology 101	197
Is There Research to Support These Claims?	198
A New Approach to Healthy Weight Loss - Lowering Leptin	201
For Every Action, There Is an Opposite and Equal Reaction	202
Eat GRAS!	203
Survival of the Fittest, not the Fattest	204
How to Make This Discovery Work for You	205
Make fat loss your goal, not weight loss	206
Customize Calculate Your Calories to Churn and Burn	207
Mifflin Equation	207
Putting it All Together - 5 Ways to Boost Your Metabolism	209

CHAPTER FOURTEEN: BREAKING THROUGH PLATEAUS: UNDERSTANDING PLATEAUS IN WEIGHT LOSS
BY JIM HOVEN, DC — **206**

Understanding Plateaus in Weight Loss	212
How Learning From the Past Creates Success In The Future	214
What Does the Body's Basal Metabolic Rate Have To Do With Weight?	215
The Top Tips To Accelerate Your Weight Loss Breakthrough	217

CHAPTER FIFTEEN:
EATING A BALANCED MEAL
BY MICHELE ASKAR, DC — 223

What are you currently doing when preparing your meals? 224
What are your goals? 224
So you may be asking yourself what is the best way for me? 225
What is the hidden secret to success? 226
Balanced Diet Meals For One Week 227
Balanced Diet – Lunch – Snack 228
Balanced Diet - Dinner Plan 229
Dr. Askar's Weight Loss Tips 231
Recipes to design a balanced meal for you 232

CHAPTER SIXTEEN: HOW STRESS AFFECTS WEIGHT LOSS
BY BRADY SCHUYLER, DC — 236

What is Stress? 242 The Role of Hormones In Stress 243
Is Your Stress Response Normal? 243 Heart and Circulation: 245
Stress's Devastating Effects 247
A Past Metaphor to Understand Stress Better 247
Three Questions to Ask Yourself 247
The Three Common Areas of Stress 247
Ask Yourself, "What is right for me?" 250
Ask, how does this apply to me? 251
How much should I strive to improve? 251
A simple philosophy is to imagine a healthy person. 252

CHAPTER SEVENTEEN: UNDERSTANDING THE NEUROTRANSMITTERS AND HORMONES THAT AFFECT WEIGHT CONTROL
BY STEVEN TROEGER, DC & DEBORAH L. TROEGER — 248

What are Neurotransmitters? 254
What do Hormones Have to Do With It? 256
Influences On Our Hormones 257
What About Serotonin and Your Adrenal Glands? 260
Can You Control Your Weight With Neurotransmitters? 262
What Can You Expect When Supplementing With Amino Acids? 263
It's To Bad We Don't have Warning Lights 266
Quick Tips For Neurotransmitters in Weight Management. 267
WHICH CARB-ADDICTED BRAIN TYPE ARE YOU? 269
Essential Nutritional Support For All Types 270

Chapter Eighteen: High Tech Solution To Weight Loss
by Patrick K. Porter, Ph.D. — 273

How is technology changing the way we use our brain?	276
How do tones create relaxation?	277
How Binaural Beats Work	278
How does light create relaxation?	279
Four Brainwave Frequencies	280
Why use light and sound together?	281
What is the secret to getting these kinds of results?	282
What are the Best Light & Sound Parameters?	282
What is the Benefit in Achieving the Alpha and Theta States?	284
What are the Benefits of Light and Sound Technology?	285

Chapter Nineteen: Recognize Hidden Thyroid Problems In Weight Loss
by Mark Lewis, DC — 287

What is the importance of the thyroid in weight loss?	288
What has caused our national health to spiral out of control?	288
What are the symptoms of an underactive thyroid?	290
The symptoms of hypothyroidism include:	290
What are the symptoms of an overactive thyroid?	292
Other symptoms include:	292
What tests are performed to diagnose a thyroid problem?	293
What causes thyroid dysfunction and why is it more common?	295
What is the importance of iodine in thyroid dysfunction?	297
Structure of Iodine	298
What is the current conventional approach?	299
What is the advantage of using a bioidentical hormone like Amour Thyroid?	300
What are some lifestyle recommendations to improve thyroid health?	301

Chapter Twenty: The Importance of Water
by Jon Steffins, DC — 303

What is The Truth about Water?	304
What Does the Research say?	305
Water is energy	306
Are You Energy Bankrupt?	307

Let's connect the water dots	*308*
Mundane to Exotic	*309*
Water… No Additives needed	*311*
Knowledge is the beginning of wisdom	*311*
Six Tips to Drinking More water	*312*

CHAPTER TWENTY-ONE: EXERCISE AND WEIGHT LOSS
BY JEFF WISDO, DC — **313**

The role of exercise in overall health	*314*
The role of exercise in weight loss	*316*
What are the best exercises for me to help with my weight loss?	*316*
Walking - The Perfect Weight Loss Exercise	*319*
My Walking Story	*320*

CHAPTER TWENTY-TWO:
ADDITIONAL RESOURCES — **322**

MEET THE AUTHORS	*323*

Dedication

This book is dedicated to you, the reader. We commend you for staying the course and seeking the truth. It was with you and your wellbeing in mind that we pulled together the wealth of knowledge within the HS HealthSource System to bring you this guide for achieving your natural weight. We ask only that you suspend your disbelief long enough to test out the tips, recipes, and meal plans in Freedom From Fat for yourself. We are confident that, once you do so, you will enjoy the same kind of energy, health, and vitality as the authors do!

Acknowledgement

Two years ago, when I started working with the HealthSource doctors to bring the behavioral repatterning component to their already successful weight loss program, I realized that I had tapped into a wellspring of knowledge on nutrition and health that needed to be shared with the millions of Americans fighting the battle of the bulge. This book is a collaboration of many, and is meant to touch the lives of as many individuals as possible. I would like to thank everyone who put their hearts and souls into this project, starting with Dr. Chris Tomshack, DC, who is not only the brains behind the formation of the HS HealthSource Chiropractic and Progressive Rehab franchise system, but also a visionary for the chiropractic field and its role in the changing world of wellness. Thanks also go out to Dr. Kevin Huffman, MD who has been a guiding light in the medical community as he campaigns for a natural solution to the obesity epidemic.

Special thanks to all the HealthSource doctors who added their brilliant insights and were dedicated to putting this work together. Dr. Richard Kearns, Dr. Chad Young, Dr. Joseph Hayes, Dr. Amanda Borre, Dr. Frank Dachtler, Dr. Brandon Pettke, Dr. Jessi Rezac, Dr. Mason Orth, Dr. Jeremy Busch, Dr. Andy Nelson, Dr. Jim Hoven, Dr. Michele Askar, Dr. Brady Schuyler, Dr. Steven Troeger, Deborah L. Troeger, Dr. Mark Lewis, Dr. Jon Steffins, Dr. Jeff Wisdo. Each of these doctors brought a special gift to this work. To see a list of their accomplishments, please go to the ìMeet the Authorsî pages in the Additional Resources Chapter in the back of the book.

Thanks go out to the Corporate Staff at HS HealthSource, with special thanks to Carrie Puhalla. Without her organizational skills, this work would likely still be in the planning stages.

In my journey of writing books over the last 20 years, I have come to rely on the talents of my family. Thankfully, I have a large family, which means I have plenty of help. I would like to acknowledge my wife, Cynthia, for her help and encouragement in putting the text together and sharing her special gift as a writer. Thanks to my sister-in law, Heidi Porter, for accepting the challenge of working with each of the authors and editing their work to be included in the book. And thanks to my brother, Michael J Porter, Jr., who served as national nutrition director for my previous company. Michael's tireless quest for the secrets to optimum health has always served to bring to light the cutting edge research and information that helps our clients take weight off and lead a healthy life.

Thanks, too, to Jason Rina, for sharing his exceptional artistic talent in the design of this book cover.

Foreword

America is facing an epidemic of excessive weight and obesity that threatens our nation. In the United States over the past two decades we've seen a doubling of adult obesity and a tripling of adolescent obesity. It's not simply a matter of our population getting larger, it's the co-morbidities associated with excessive weight such as diabetes, heart disease, strokes, cancers, liver disease, respiratory disease as well as a plethora of other medical conditions that is threatening our very existence. For the first time in recorded history, our children's generation will live shorter lives than their parents due to these chronic diseases associated with excessive weight. We're seeing an epidemic of Type 2 diabetes in the US that is directly related to the obesity epidemic. We're seeing rising rates of cancer and heart disease as a result of the obesity epidemic, and it's not just the adult population that is suffering from obesity related disease.

There is debate about the etiology of this epidemic, from excessive portion sizes, to changes in macro and micro nutrient composition of our foods, to the explosive growth of fast foods, to dramatic decreases in our daily physical activity. Regardless of the cause of this epidemic, there should be no debate as to the treatment. The treatment of our obesity epidemic will require an army of healthcare providers armed with knowledge of the disease process, treatment options, and a willingness to devote their time and professional expertise to battling this epidemic.

Where will that army come from? The medical community has been sitting on the sidelines watching this epidemic grow and strangle our nation's health and healthcare budgets, as tens of millions of Americans are turned away from conventional medical interventions and ultimately finding themselves in the hands of commercial weight loss centers or utilizing unproven and potentially dangerous fad diet products.

It's understandable in today's healthcare system why the established medical community has failed to address this obesity epidemic. A recent study reveals that only 20 of 112 medical colleges surveyed offered a single nutrition class, and none offered a bariatric (medical weight management) class. Our traditional allopathic and osteopathic training falls short in the basic science of nutrition, behavior, and exercise. Our healthcare system, which is designed upon a platform of addressing acute care issues only and hence ignoring preventive and wellness issues, discourages physicians from addressing the complete and time-consuming issues that surround obesity care.

There is hope, however, in a healthcare community whose roots are well imbedded in the science of nutrition, exercise, and behavior modification. These are physicians who are not only trained in these core sciences but who have the expertise, staffing, and experience in managing chronic healthcare issues such as obesity. They are physicians who also understand and practice prevention and wellness medicine. I am speaking of the *chiropractic community*, physicians who are well positioned to become our nation's warriors in this battle with obesity.

How do we engage these physicians who seem best suited to address this disease? That was a question that I had been grappling with for several years until I met Dr. Chris Tomshack, a chiropractic physician and entrepreneur who shared my vision of recruiting the chiropractic community into the war on obesity, but who was able to back his vision with a network of chiropractic physicians from coast to coast.

Dr Tomshack had built a successful network of chiropractic physicians through his national HealthSource™ business to address chiropractic and rehab issues, and he has now turned his efforts toward training and supporting this national network of physicians into the army of healthcare providers we need to wage war on obesity. Dr. Tomshack has assembled physicians, nutritionists, exercise experts, psychologists, and behaviorists to help train and support this weight management army.

In this exciting new book, you'll hear from some of these experts. In this well-written, concise and practical handbook you'll learn the role macro and micro nutrients play in obesity and obesity management, you'll have an opportunity to review the science behind good fats and bad fats, carbohydrates, insulin, sugars, the glycemic index, sugar substitutes, the role protein plays in weight management. and the importance of fiber and water in weight loss. There are great examples of healthy meal planning from chiropractic physicians with years of experience in treating overweight and obese patients. These doctors utilize nutritional science principles and put that science into practical solutions. They also look at the role of exercise in weight loss and weight maintenance.

You'll learn the secret power of detoxifying for weight loss, how natural enzymes, the master metabolic regulator, the thyroid, and our own immune system affect our weight. The science of stress, brain neurotransmitters, and hormones are discussed and practical advice is given on how to boost metabolism and break through those difficult and frustrating weight loss plateaus.

Throughout the text, you'll find clearly defined chapters that go beyond simple weight loss and to the core of wellness such a how acid/base and pH impacts health, the importance of oxygen and the lymphatic system in our ability to reach optimal health, how to reverse the aging process, and the detrimental effects of inflammation on the human body.

A topic very rarely covered in a book on weight management is that of how we think and act in relation to our weight. Dr. Patrick Porter, a noted expert on mind-based weight loss and wellness, shares his insightful understanding of how patients visualize their health status, and how utilizing creative visualization and relaxation (CVR) together can create breakthroughs by changing beliefs about weight and weight loss and alleviating the stress effect. Finally, Dr. Porter discusses the advancements that have been made in behavior therapies through technologic breakthroughs and how such technologies, such as light/sound/CVR combinations, have created opportunities for overweight patients to finally succeed at losing weight and keeping it weight off.

  I applaud Dr. Tomshack and his colleagues at HealthSource for developing the weight management guidelines for chiropractic physicians; it represents just one of many steps he has taken to fulfill his vision of creating an army of physicians that will take back our nation's health and finally reverse this epidemic of obesity that we face in America today. I am thrilled that he teamed up with Dr. Porter to write this book for those who are fighting the battle at a personal level. I also strongly encourage any and all physicians to read this insightful and practical book and apply the principles to help their patients lose weight, improve health, and take back control of their lives.

Dr. Kevin Huffman
American Bariatric Consultants
Vermilion, Ohio

Dr. Huffman is a board certified bariatric medical physician. He has been instrumental in training and educating US physicians in the art and science of bariatric medicine for over two decades. A leading medical authority on obesity and its metabolic diseases, he has trained and mentored hundreds of physicians, nurses, dieticians, exercise specialists, and behaviorists as bariatric educator for the American Society of Bariatric Physicians, the American Board of Bariatric Medicine, the Obesity Society, and the American Society for Metabolic and Bariatric Surgery.

Introduction

Please, not another weight loss book! If this is your first impression, that's okay. Take a walk down the health aisle at any book store or peruse the offerings online, and you'll be inundated and overwhelmed with the never ending offerings of weight loss books available for the desperate dieter's consumption.

Indulge me here for a minute. What are most of these books about? You've got it, mostly fad diets and wild, outlandish claims of losing all the weight you want to lose while still eating vast amounts of cherry pie. Let's get real here. This book is fundamentally different from the great majority of weight loss books available today. When it comes to real, usable information, it's pretty darn difficult to find a weight loss book that gives you the information—the truth—you need to make positive, long-term weight loss a real possibility. This is the book that has the information you crave. That's why it was written.

So let's forget the fad, celebrity diets. Forget about counting calories. Forget about keeping track of points. Points for this and points for that...all you end up doing is focusing so much on food that you can't get food out of your mind! These are not the ingredients for a long-term weight loss solution. But you'll get the secret to lasting weight loss success within these pages.

What about diet pills? Don't they work? Let me tell you this. Of the many thousands of patients I treated over the years, I never met one person who kept the weight off when they used unhealthy diet pills. Think back to the 90's. Remember PhenFen? It was the pharmaceutical weight loss cocktail that ended with heart valve damage for thousands of users and eventual legal damages to the tune of $13 billion. Yes, it was pulled from the market, but too late for many who were permanently injured from those little pills in which they had placed so much hope. Pills are not the answer, not by a long shot.

So this book was written for all of you who are fed up with those ridiculous diets and empty promises from some huckster trying to sell books or products, and unhealthy advice from the uninformed or easily persuaded. This book is designed to give you relevant information so that YOU can lose your excess pounds and keep them off, long term. Certainly you've learned that it can be more dangerous to lose weight, gain it back, lose it, and gain it back yet again than to just stay overweight, right? Let's break that cycle. Let's do it right. Let's do it in a healthy manner.

If losing weight were as simple as taking a pill or counting calories or counting points, there wouldn't be an obesity epidemic in America. We know this because Americans are getting fatter every year. Counting points or calories and popping pills aren't helping. This book reveals, to many of you for the very first time, the information others are afraid to give you. They're scared to tell you the truth because then they can't sell their sham diets. It would expose them for what they really are, which is contrary to their mission. And their mission is to separate you from your cash, pure and simple.

Consulting with patients who were always counting points and calories revealed a certain pattern to me. And the pattern is exhibited by a complete obsession with food due to the fact that you must be counting and analyzing your food intake all day long. It's counter productive. What we think about we bring about. And if we focus on food all day, it becomes an obsession, an obsession you can't defeat. And sooner or later you lose the battle and the pounds come piling back. This is no way to live your life. Let's learn how to lose weight the right way, without obsession and without heartache.

This book is also designed to take you step by step into the world of healthy weight loss. It's a world that, once you enter, you'll no longer fall prey to the fad diet mongers of the world. And this is because you'll have the information necessary to construct and follow a healthy, long-term solution in the battle of the bulge.

In this book we'll teach you things you had no idea are so vitally important. Things like acid/base balance, oxygenation, detoxification, body chemistry, protein importance, sugar awareness, fiber mastery, the role of enzymes, how stress affects weight loss and on and on. The goal here is not to turn you into a doctor or a weight loss fanatic. It's to give you the correct information so that you can have an understanding of why you've likely failed on many diets before. Many times, it's not your fault. How can you be expected to follow a fatally flawed diet in the first place? How can you be expected to lose weight and keep it off on an inherently unhealthy concoction of food and supplements? The missing link was information. This book delivers that information in a clear, concise, readable format. It's a format you can digest.

    I suggest you read one chapter a day until finished. Then it's time for action. It's time for real, sustainable weight loss.

    Today, the weight loss industry is doing about $60 billion a year. Most of that money might as well be flushed down the toilet each and every year, quickly replaced by new money. And the weight loss companies love it. They love it because the failure rate with diets is so ridiculously high; they are just about guaranteed to get you back as a repeat customer. Now that's a sustainable business.

    I'm telling you that you don't have to participate in the classic weight loss industry. There will be no need. Once you have the correct, useable information, you can simply opt out of this predatory industry. Go ahead and opt out for life. Your bank account will thank you. Your heirs will thank you. You will thank you.

    I'm the CEO of the world's largest chiropractic, rehab and weight loss franchise company. We treat hundreds of thousands of patients across this great country. The most common deterrent to good health that we encounter is the obesity epidemic. Our patients are suffering from diabetes, high blood pressure, chronic fatigue, and painful joints in ever increasing numbers. With that reason in mind, the doctors of HealthSource got together to write this book. You can read it and use the information to help you lose your weight for life, or you can choose to do nothing. That's your right. Some of you may decide you need additional help getting started. That's fine, too. That's why we're here.

Before you dig into this book much further, I encourage you to find a highlighter or pen so that you can mark up the book as you go. Highlight or underline what you deem to be the most important points for you, so that you can find them easier as you reference this book. Because it's time now for you to arm yourself with good, solid, healthy information to help you lose that extra weight and keep it off. And if you encounter something you don't quite understand, don't fret. You can contact my company and ask us any questions you have. And you can do this for free. Simply email us at questions@healthsourcechiro.com. You can also look us up on the web at www.healthsourcesuccess.com. There is a forum where you can pose questions as well. I encourage you to take us up on this offer.

So dispose of those diet pills, throw away the fad diet books, and get ready to learn what you've been missing. Each chapter is designed to give you one more of the integral building blocks of long term, safe, healthy weight loss. A lot has been written about these building blocks, but never before in a concise format like *Freedom from Fat* offers you. We've put it in simple to understand language that you can start using for your benefit today.

Lastly, from time to time you may make a mistake while losing and keeping off your weight. That's not the time to give up or to fall into negative thoughts. Hey, you're human, right? Just get back up on the horse and keep going forward. I'm a big proponent of a cheat day. In my life, that's Saturday. My family actually has a "Saturday ice cream fest," where we sit down and have some ice cream together—real ice cream, too! Life shouldn't be so rigid that we stop enjoying it. It must be fluid, dynamic and fun. Otherwise, what's the use? Knowing that you can have fun with food while losing weight—well, it just makes this whole weight loss thing doable.

So now it's your turn. Grab the highlighter and dig into chapter one. You're not alone.

CHAPTER ONE

The Acid/Base Balance
Richard Kearns, DC

ACID/BASE BALANCE
by Richard Kearns, DC

The College Discovery That Changed My Life

I started researching Acid/Base balance a few years back while in college. I was 20 years old, had acid reflux, irritable bowel syndrome; and I was told I was on the verge of a stomach ulcer. When I had the testing done to determine to what extent the damage was, I was essentially told that I had way too much acid in my stomach and would have to be on medication the rest of my life. At the age of 20, I didn't like that idea. Since I plan on living for quite some time, I began to look at ways these conditions occur and why and what to do to either decrease the severity of the symptoms or eliminate them entirely. Through my digging around I came across a lot of good information and some information that wasn't as good.

This chapter is going to discuss the Acid/Base Balance of the body and how it plays a role in weight loss, as well as other effects it has on the body in an easy to follow manner. Before we begin, I want to just clarify the difference between an acid and base--a little throwback to chemistry class--without getting too scientific. The determination of whether something is an acid or acidic and a base or basic depends on the pH scale.

This scale goes from 0 to 14. On the scale, the lower the number the more acidic something is. The higher the number, the more basic it is. A pH of 7 is considered neutral-

-neither acidic or basic. It's the midline. Our bodies work hard to maintain a certain pH level. For example, the pH of our blood must be in the range of 7.35 – 7.45, slightly basic. The pH of urine is 6.0-6.5, stomach acid is 2.0, saliva is 6.0-7.4. The point is that different parts and fluids of the body have different pH levels and the blood levels have a narrow range to maintain. There are different ways to check where your body stands.

How To Check Your pH

The easiest way to check your body's pH is to get pH strips from your local health food store. Some drug stores may also carry them. These will either be for your urine or saliva. You either insert the pH strip into your urine stream or on your tongue and then compare it to a color chart they come with. Based on the test strip reading, you can then tell if you are in a more acidic state or basic state. Another way to check pH is either a blood test and/or a urinalysis. However, these tests need to be ordered by your physician, and lets face it, unless you are checking for other things in your blood or urine it's not going to be economical to just test for pH.

Most of the problems in our bodies related to health and weight are related to having too much acid flowing through the body. There are some symptoms and conditions that may indicate if you are too acidic. They include, but are not limited to:

- Cardiovascular damage, including the constriction of blood vessels and the reduction of oxygen.
- Weight gain, obesity and diabetes.
- Bladder and kidney conditions, including kidney stones.
- Immune deficiency.
- Acceleration of free radical damage, possibly contributing to cancerous mutations.
- Hormone concerns.
- Premature aging.
- Osteoporosis; weak, brittle bones, hip fractures and bone spurs.
- Joint pain, aching muscles and lactic acid buildup.
- Low energy and chronic fatigue.
- Slow digestion and elimination.
- Yeast/fungal overgrowth.

How Do Symptoms Develop From Too Much Acid?

I'm going to give you a brief explanation so you have an understanding of how the body deals with acids and bases. The research started way back in 1914, so this concept isn't exactly new. Loren Cordain, PhD was a professor and researcher at Colorado State University, Fort Collins, in the department of health and exercise science. Dr. Cordain did early research on acid-yielding and base-yielding foods. To sum things up, he found that after digestion occurs, all the food reports to the kidneys as either acidic or basic.

Now the significance of this is that one of the kidney's

jobs is to balance the fluids of the body and maintain a relatively neutral pH--preferably slightly basic. When acidic foods lower the body's pH, the kidneys do what they can to buffer the acidity. Your bones release calcium and magnesium to reestablish the basic nature of the body. The muscles break down and produce ammonia, which is strongly basic. When everything is said and done, your bone mineral and broken down muscle gets excreted into the urine. Now short term, this is okay for your body. However, long term acidity from the diet breaks the bones and muscles down further and further and we end up with decreased bone mass and decreased strength, which given enough time will cause the conditions listed above--to name just a few.

The main reason all of the above happens or can happen is all based on what the average American diet entails. It consists mainly of lots of beef, eggs, soda pop, sweet sugary foods and snacks, and dairy and too little of our green leafy veggies, fruits, and other colorful veggies. I, myself, grew up with parents who didn't like the taste of a lot of fruits or vegetable.

We were a typical meat and potatoes family for sure. The only fruits and veggies we ate in my house were corn, apples, oranges and the occasional salad with iceberg lettuce. Looking back, it's no wonder I was on the verge of an ulcer at the age of 20!

Now let's look at the pH of some common substances and foods a bit further.

Substance	pH	Acid/Base
Sodium Hydroxide	14.0	Base
Lye	13.0	Base
Ammonia	11.0	Base
Milk of Magnesia	10.5	Base
Baking Soda	8.3	Base
Human blood	7.4	Base
PURE Water	7.0	Neutral
Milk	6.6	Acid
Tomatoes	4.5	Acid
Wine and Beer	4.0	Acid
Apples	3.0	Acid
Vinegar	2.2	Acid
Lemon Juice	2.0	Acid
Battery Acid	1.0	Acid
Hydrochloric Acid	0.0	Acid

Those are the pH's of some substances and foods. I know this is a book on weight loss, but I wanted you to have some frame of reference for how acidic some foods can be compared to things we already know are acidic or basic.

The point is that even though some of the foods listed above are acidic to start, after digestion they leave a basic residue, or are base-yielding.

Let's give you a couple lists of both acid and base-yielding foods. These are very limited lists just to give you an idea of the types of foods on each list.

Acid-Yielding Foods

Spaghetti	Peanuts	Walnuts
Corn Flakes	Whole Wheat Bread	
Eggs	White Rice	Rolled Oats
Salami	Rye Bread	Brown Rice
Lunch Meats	White Bread	Cottage Cheese
Liver	Whole Milk	Gouda Cheese Cod
Lentils	Hard Cheese	Herring
Beef	Chicken	Processes Cheeses (soft)
Pork	Trout	Parmesan Cheese

Base-Yielding Foods

Apricots	Cucumbers	Tomatoes
Kiwifruit	Green Peppers	Eggplant
Cherries	Broccoli	Lettuce (greener the better)
Bananas	Cauliflower	Green Beans
Strawberries	Zucchini	Onions
Peaches	Carrots	Mushrooms
Oranges	Celery	Mineral Water
Lemon Juice	Watermelon	Spinach
Pears	Apples	Raisins
Pineapples	Peaches	Dates

Do you notice anything about the base-yielding foods compared to the acid-forming foods?

Fruits and vegetables are all base-yielding unless they are marinated or pickled in some manner. A further note is that any food that is processed in any manner affects how it is processed by the body. For example, apples and oranges--acidic to start--are basic by the time they are digested. Now let's juice them, throw in some white processed sugar to sweeten them up some more, maybe add some coloring, and other preservatives.

How do you think your body will process it now? If you guessed acidic, you are right on. The reason for this is that when you add all the extras to a pure fruit or vegetable, our bodies barely recognize anything healthy in it. Store bought bottles of juices, whether veggie or fruit, having been processed, affects the way it is digested by your body as well.

If you choose to juice them yourself, the best method is to simply just juice and don't add anything to it to sweeten it up; and remember, because you aren't adding all those preservatives, fresh juices would have to be consumed soon after juicing while the enzymes, antioxidants, and other good stuff are still available for proper use by your body.

White sugar and white flour are acid-yielding substances as well; and they seem to be in anything processed. For those of you who love or "need" your morning coffee, guess what? That turns into acid as well; and if you think using artificial sweeteners will decrease the acidity because you are not using white sugar, think again. Nutrasweet, Equal, and aspartame just to name a few are all acid forming substances. A lot of drugs that people use are acid forming as well.

Several things can occur and proliferate in an acidic body. There are bacteria, yeasts (candida mainly) and fungi that show up in acidic bodies. They are attracted to acidic environments. I have seen in past research where bacteria, yeasts, and fungi may cause the body to crave sweets and sugars, which leads to more acid deposits in the body. More so, these can lead to further problems with other conditions-- urinary tract infections, yeast infections, and fungal infections such as athletes foot, just to name a few.

What Role Does Stress Play?

Another factor that can lead to an acidic body environment is high levels of stress, both physical or emotional. The physical component stems from too much exercise--believe it or not, some people exercise too much--and highly physical jobs at work and at home. When you do physical activity beyond what you normally do, your muscles release Lactic Acid, which, you guessed it, is an acid. This serves as a protective mechanism initially. It stops you from overworking your muscles.

When you rest between your sets, or workouts, or job, the body does what it can to reduce and/or get rid of the excess lactic acid. However, when you keep working and working and working above and beyond what your body is capable of recovering from fully, leading to increased acid in the muscles. This then leads to muscle soreness, trigger points, spasms, and pain for some.

The emotional aspect of stress causes the body to release a hormone called Cortisol. Cortisol is also released in conjunction with Lactic Acid during physical stress. Cortisol is released from the adrenal glands, which sit on top of the kidneys. It is released to attempt to help us handle stress. When it comes to weight, especially, it is believed to have a huge (no pun intended) effect on weight gain/loss. Cortisol does a few different functions in the body that can affect acidity and weight gain.

When Cortisol is released, it increases the body's blood sugar, increases blood pressure, and suppresses your body's immune system. This is all part of the body's fight or flight system, which is essential to survival; however, long term, this becomes a problem. If you refer back to the symptoms/conditions caused by too much acid in the body, you will be able to see the connection to all of this. Fight or flight causes the body to release Cortisol and adrenaline in the body. In addition to that, your pupils dilate, thinking improves, lungs breath easier, digestion virtually ceases, and our appetite suppresses. Essential actions when you come face to face with a bear or lion--but how often does that happen? If it's happening on a daily basis due to high stress from your boss, your spouse or significant other, or working out excessively, it's not good.

How this all works is that when Cortisol is released it triggers an increase in blood glucose (blood sugar) by converting glucose from protein. Muscle is made up of protein. That is where the muscle is broken down. So muscle breaks down and converts to glucose, which can lead to an increase in release of insulin in the body. Insulin's job is to keep blood sugar levels stable.

So if there is an increase or a spike in blood sugar, insulin will convert glucose to fat stores. Then when the stress goes away or minimizes, adrenaline returns to normal, but Cortisol will linger on to help balance the body further. One way it balances out is that it will increase your appetite after the stress is gone to restore all the reserves you lost due to the stress, which can lead to overeating further. The significance of this is in the fact that everyday stress is triggering Cortisol release, hence our appetites go up. Our appetites going up leads to increased food intake, which leads to increased weight.

The one area of the body believed to be affected by high Cortisol levels is the belly. The belly is believed to be the area where all the fat is stored as a result of Cortisol. If this is happening on a daily basis, can you understand how weight gain as well as other conditions are affected? This is another reason our society seems to be gaining more and more weight--most people are under a lot more stress daily than they have ever been in the past. We all believed that technology was supposed to make our lives easier.

As we are beginning to understand, though, the better technology gets, the more we feel we have to get done on a daily basis. Whether it is self induced or caused by the outside influences in our lives, either way we live in a constant barrage of stress after stress.

Tips for Keeping Your pH at an Optimal Level

Tip #1 First things first. To find out what your pH is, go get some pH strips. You can find them online or at you local health food store or drug store.

Tip #2 Evaluate what you eat and compare it to the lists given. Eat more foods in the lists that are base-yielding. Get rid of drinks that increase acids in the body, i.e. soda pop, beer, wine and sugary drinks.

Tip #3 Increase your pure water intake along with natural fruit and vegetable juices. To further do that with water, one of the best things you can do is start your day off first thing with lemon water. Just squeeze a lemon into a tall glass of water to get the body cleansing right away.

Tip #4 Manage your stress levels as best you can. One way is by using the BRD (Behavioral Repatterning Device) discussed in this book.

Tip #5 Exercise moderately both resistance and aerobic--again discussed later in this book.

I am not saying you have to avoid all your favorite foods forever. Making better choices for yourself with good wholesome foods and water goes a long way, so when you do consume your favorite foods, they don't make your body acidic. You may very likely even notice a change in any aches/pains or condition you are currently experiencing. Leading to increase energy levels and a better life overall.

There are also plenty of supplements that can be taken to help with increasing your pH levels, but I would highly recommend starting with what we've talked about thus far before supplementing, especially if you want to lose weight and keep it off. This is only one factor of many to losing weight, but first you have to make a decision to change, then follow the steps consistently to doing so. If you follow the same path as you have been, you won't get far. Good luck on your journey to a new life and a new you.

> *"Of all the self-fulfilling prophecies in our culture, the assumption that aging means decline and poor health is probably the deadliest."*
> **Marilyn Ferguson, The Aquarian Conspiracy, 1980**

CHAPTER TWO

Oxygen's Role In Weight Loss
Chad Young, DC

Oxygen's Role in Weight Loss
By Chad Young, DC

What is the Lymphatic System and Why is it Important?

Many people aren't aware of it, but a healthy body depends on the Lymphatic System. It is a "second" circulatory system that is four times larger than the circulatory system. It is the body's defense system that rids the body of debris including fats, toxins, infections and viruses--carrying this debris away from the cells to enhance our total health.

The lymphatic system is a series of vessels that transport waste products and foreign invaders through the interstitial fluid. The interstitial fluid is important in maintaining cells and tissues. As it travels through the lymphatic system it is called lymph fluid. This is a colorless fluid that carries white blood cells to fight viruses and bacteria. It also contains salt, protein, glucose and urea.

Every cell in the body has a sodium potassium pump in it that generates electricity, which is power. Everywhere you have a blood vessel going through your body you have a corresponding lymph vessel going side by side, with cells running in between. The purpose of the lymphatic vessels is to pull out all the dead cells, poisons and excess water from the spaces around the cells. This is called a dry state. The cells have to be kept in a dry state to get oxygen from the blood vessels.

As you can see, the lymphatic system is very important to our overall health. However, this system has serious limitations, because unlike the circulatory system, it has no pump to help it carry out these tasks. This system must rely on us. We are responsible for its maintenance and for keeping it running properly. If we don't maintain proper diet and exercise the lymphatic system will fail to function properly, causing weight gain, swelling and disease.

Lymphedema and Our Weight

One of the most serious problems associated with an improperly functioning lymphatic system is lymphedema, also known as lymphatic obstruction. This is a condition of localized fluid retention and tissue swelling caused by a compromised lymphatic system. When this occurs, there is an accumulation of lymphatic fluid in the tissues of the body and swelling results.

Symptoms can include severe fatigue, a heavy swollen limb or localized fluid accumulation in other body areas including the head or neck, discoloration of the skin overlying the lymphedema and eventually deformity. If you suspect this condition, consult your doctor to check for obstructions in the lymphatic system.

Lymphedema may be inherited or caused by injury to the lymphatic vessels. It is most frequently seen after lymph node dissection, surgery or radiation therapy. It may also be associated with accidents, certain diseases or problems that inhibit the lymphatic system from functioning properly. It can also be caused by compromising the lymphatic system resulting from cellulitis.

Lymphedema may be present at birth, develop during puberty or not become apparent until adulthood. In women it is most prevalent in the upper limbs after breast cancer surgery or lymph node dissection. It can also occur in the lower limbs or groin after surgery for colon, ovarian or uterine cancer in which removal of the lymph nodes was required. In men, lower limb lymphedema is most common, occurring in one or both legs and can occur after surgery for prostate, colon or testicular cancer where lymph notes were removed or damaged.

Another cause of lymphedema is carrying excess weight. The extra weight in our bodies can press down on the lymphatic vessels so the fluid can't be moved out properly; hence, swelling in areas of the body. Later on in this chapter, we'll discuss how to correct this problem and keep the lymphatic system running smoothly to assist in your overall health and maintaining your weight.

Oxygen--the Fountain of Youth?

Many of us taking breathing for granted. We do it thousands of times per day without consciously thinking about it, but how does oxygen relate to our lymphatic system and a healthy body? Increasing oxygen levels in the blood stream increases energy by burning more calories. I like to compare our bodies to a car engine. You can put the best gasoline in the world in the tank, but if you're not getting oxygen to the gasoline, it's not going to burn. In humans, you can eat a great, nutritious meal, but if you're not pumping new oxygen into your body, you are not going to burn calories the way you need to burn them for optimal health. The more oxygen you get, the quicker you're going to get rid of old cells and produce new ones.

Now, think of how oxygen travels through the body--through the circulatory system. It's a highway of sorts. The highway delivers oxygen all throughout the body. The lymphatic system is there to protect your body from harmful toxins--but how does it get to these toxins? Through the circulatory system. It needs the circulatory system to bring the intruders to it and send its warriors out to fight infections.

How do we get more oxygen into our bodies? The obvious answer is through exercise. You have two types of exercise--weight lifting and cardio. Cardio is going to be more efficient at getting oxygen into the blood stream. Also, the movement of cardio exercise helps assist in moving the lymphatic system.

Weight lifting is going to create new muscle, which will help burn more calories and it also actually drives calcium into the bones--a great thing for women--to help prevent osteoporosis. You need a good balance of both types of exercise to keep your motor running efficiently. And, again, the more oxygen in your body the more efficiently the cardiovascular system operates and the more efficiently the lymphatic system works as well. For more information on exercise, you can refer to Chapter 21 of this book.

Helping the Lymphatic System Perform at its Peak

Now that we know what the lymphatic system is and how it functions in our body, what can we do to ensure that we do all that we can to help it along? Well, obviously fueling the body with the right nutrients is very important, but there are other ways to keep the lymphatic system running in peak condition. The body needs to move. The lymph system works with each cell in the body, bringing nutrients to the cell and taking waste products away. Unlike blood, which is pumped by the heart, the lymphatic system is totally dependent on movement to work properly.

One of those methods is massage. As we talked about earlier, the lymphatic system doesn't have a heart pumping it around. The movement of the fluid in the lymphatic system is from muscles pushing on the vessels, causing the fluid to move forward in the vessel. With massage you actually have somebody or something pressing on the body, pressing on the vessel, moving the fluid through the lymphatic system. You can hire a massage therapist to do this--which is great--but it can get costly.

In my office we use a Panasonic massage chair. It's basically doing the same thing as a massage therapist. You get massage, you get muscle work, you're moving the lymphatic system. That helps get new oxygen to the muscles and tissues. The difference is, once you buy a massage chair, you have it for use every day--and the whole family can benefit from its use. A massage a day can stimulate the release of ATP (adenosine triphosphate) the molecules from which all cells derive energy; increases phagocytosis (encapsulating and eliminating pathogens and debris); increases circulatory function to move nutrients, gases and wastes to and from cells--fighting disease to maintain homeostasis; stimulates the production of collagen, thus reducing pain and inflammation; aides in tissue regeneration, the repair process of cells and much more.

The massage chair is but one option for moving the lymphatic system. Another option is using what is called a vibration plate. This is a plate you stand or sit on that vibrates your entire body. This causes the muscles and tissues in the body to actually start to move, moving every cell in your body. The vibration plate helps burn fat and cellulite, tones and tightens skin, increases serotonin levels, decreases joint pain, and increases flexibility and balance. These are available online for about $199 to thousands of dollars depending on what you choose. When you use these vibration plates, you can actually feel your temperature rising. When your temperature rises, you're burning calories.

A surprising way to help our lymphatic system operate more effectively in our body is to be careful of the types of clothing we choose. Any clothing that is tight against the skin restricts lymphatic flow. Bras with under wires are particularly harmful in restricting the lymphatic flow in the breast area.

Rebounding

Another great way to help move the lymphatic system is rebounding. It's another form of exercise that's similar to vibration. You use a small trampoline that can be adjusted to add varying amounts of resistance and tension. Once again, you're moving up and down but you're not just moving one body part. You're moving the entire body. Every time you bounce up you're contracting leg muscles which push against the lymphatic vessels, moving the lymphatic fluid through the body. The main lymph vessels run up the legs, arms and through the torso. This is why the vertical movement of rebounding is so effective at moving the fluid. Remember, as you continue jumping, you also breathe harder, increasing the amount of oxygen that you put into your system.

To prove my point, take a look at some of the quotes from a 1979 study done by NASA using a rebounder.

"Rebound Exercise is the most efficient, effective form of exercise yet devised by man." A. Carter summarized a NASA study in 1979, a study which **NASA published in 1980 in the Journal of Applied Physiology.**

NASA says, *"...for similar levels of heart rate and oxygen consumption, the magnitude of the bio mechanical stimuli is greater with jumping on a trampoline than with running, a finding that might help identify acceleration parameters needed for the design of remedial procedures to avert deconditioning in persons exposed to weightlessness. "*

When rebounding, three natural forces are at work: gravity, acceleration and deceleration. In the up and down movement of bouncing, your body is subjected to these three forces and each time you bounce into the mat (at its deepest point) your body comes into a G-force (Gravity force) of two to three.

As a consequence, literally each cell of your body experiences a G-Force which is two or three times stronger than normal. It is as if your weight would double or triple for a fraction of a second when you hit the deepest point of the Rebounder mat. This exposure to a higher G-Force is what strengthens the body; and as it is only for a fraction of a second, this does not fatigue the body. During the movement up to the highest point of your bounce, you come to nearly weightlessness and your body can relax completely.

Some important things to remember about rebounding are:
- Increases the capacity for respiration
- Circulates more oxygen to the tissues
- Causes muscles to perform the work of moving fluids through the body
- Aids in lymphatic circulation
- Strengthens the heart
- Stimulates metabolism
- Improves coordination
- Curtails fatigue
- Helps offset osteoporosis
- Helps balance blood pressure
- Activates the removal of toxins through the lymphatic system
- Improves concentration and memory

Rebounders are a relatively inexpensive way to reap all sorts of health benefits. They can run from $29 to $400 and are available at almost any sports store right down to your local Wal-Mart.

If you are one of those people who experience problems with knees or ankles, you can get some of the same benefits

CHAPTER 2 | OXYGENATING THE BODY – THE LYMPHATIC SYSTEM

of rebounding without the jump. In these cases, our office recommends using a yoga ball or balance ball. These balls can offer some of the benefits of rebounding, as well as working on posture, proprioception and balance. They help build the core muscles and help tone and tighten while losing weight. These are readily available and can be used almost anywhere.

Now that you have read all about the lymphatic system and oxygenating the body, can you really afford to ignore how important it is to your overall health and your weight loss goals? I don't think so. When I'm working with someone in my office, obviously I work on nutrition with them but the secondary problem is they're usually not moving enough. I would recommend starting off with simple walking--up to what you can tolerate. For some people this may only be a quarter of a mile a day. For some people it may be a mile or more a day. The point is to start moving.

I also like to show my patients things they can do when they're not exercising. When they're just going about their daily routine, there are so many things that could be done to enhance health. Get a massage chair and use it while watching TV. Even a hand held massager would be beneficial to use if you can't get a massage chair. That way your muscles are actually moving even during your down time. This also takes care of moving blood and lymphatic fluid in the body. You are taking care of trigger points that can cause balance issues in the body. There are many, many benefits to massage.

We also recommend using the vibration plate. They can be used while washing dishes or cooking or reading a book. They're portable and can be used all over the house. You can use the yoga ball or balance ball. Those are great to use while watching TV. Studies show that you burn more calories than sitting in your armchair and they are also great for working on balance and building core muscles.

In my office, we stress that you get moving at least three

times a day. Now, before you panic wondering how on earth you'd manage that, think about your day carefully. What are you doing in the morning routine? Can you get up twenty minutes earlier to fit in some exercise? Most of us can.

Do you have a lunch break that you can fit in a few minutes of walking? Most of us can. We don't need to spend an entire hour eating. Cut that time in half and you have plenty of time to get moving. The evening generally holds plenty of time for a few minutes of exercise. We just have to realize how important it is and do it. Even if you move for just a few minutes, that's better than nothing as far as the lymphatic system is concerned.

There you have it. By learning to keep your lymphatic system healthy and performing its job, you can put your overall health on "auto pilot." By staying healthy you will be more active and burn more calories. A healthy, lymphatic system will prevent swelling, edema, and water retention. This makes weight loss a much easier process.

> *"We lift ourselves by our thought,*
> *we climb upon our vision of ourselves.*
> *If you want to enlarge your life,*
> *you must first enlarge your thought of it and of yourself.*
> *Hold the ideal of yourself as you long to be,*
> *always, everywhere -*
> *your ideal of what you long to attain -*
> *the ideal of health, efficiency, success."*
> **Orison Swett Marden (1850 - 1924)**

CHAPTER THREE

Detoxifying the Body and Weight Loss
by Joseph Hayes, DC

The Secret Power of Detoxifying For Weight Loss
Dr. Joseph Hayes

The concept of detoxification was, until now, not often associated with weight loss. People would just start the next fad diet without preparing their bodies for the detox to come. I, personally, would not start any weight loss program without a detox first.

Preparing Your Body is Key to Weight Loss

If your goal is to take weight off and then keep it off, your first step has to be to start a detox program so your body can handle it. How are you going to lose weight more efficiently and keep it off if you are toxic? When you start your weight loss with out a cleanse program, you will only be compounding the toxins that are present in your body, which can have you feeling sluggish. Without energy, you will end up stopping your weight loss. You will only continue the cycle that had you pick up this book in the first place.

The Natural Side Benefit is Weight Loss

I would never have a patient start a detox program for the weight loss benefit alone. However, I would also never have patients start a weight loss program without detoxifying first. Health is a journey and weight loss is not the permanent goal. Maintaining your health at your proper weight is. This is why I train all my patients to make health a part of that journey. You are about to learn how your body can rise to the challenge of health in today's toxic world by not compromising from the start.

My journey started with a cancer scare. I had wanted to get my cholesterol checked, had a routine blood test and waited for what I knew would be a poor report. High cholesterol runs in my family. I had scared quite a few clinics with my results in years past. I was surprised when the doctor wouldn't look me in the eyes when I returned for my follow up. My liver enzymes were so high, it was a shoe-in, I had the big CA. Cut to the chase-- no cancer. Oh, then it must be hepatitis. No, not hep. It must be cirrhosis.

No, not cirrhosis. Then it must be--and the list went on until I finally found out what was wrong with me. It was discovered that I had poisoned myself while fueling my own airplane. I had also worked around aircraft for most of my college and grad school jobs, so possibly I had been exposed to other environmental toxins. My plane was an older one and I was very careful not to spill fuel on the wings. Standing above and watching the fuel go in was good for cleanliness and bad for my liver.

My Detox Journey

I read as much as I could on detoxification and started on the most typical of current detoxes. My girlfriend claimed I turned orange from all the carrot juice, but slowly and painfully my liver enzyme returned to normal. I was healthy again, but the road had been a long and difficult one. As I continued to read and study, I found that most of my difficulty with detoxification revolved around harming my body while I was trying to help it.

There is something spoken about while detoxing called a *health crisis*. I have now learned that this is more about crisis than health. You see, while I was clearing my body and life of all the free radicals, I was damaging myself by not allowing the free radicals to bind to something. Also, I was unaware of how my liver was responding to a restrictive diet.

What role does the liver play?

The liver is the main detoxifier of the body. However, it needs its own fuel to continue the process. I was shocked to find out the role that protein played in detoxification. By going on a restrictive diet that allowed most of my body to clean itself, I was shutting down the healing and purification process of the liver. The question was: How to keep the liver functioning while clearing the rest of the body?

I was introduced to a health product through a friend who had been practicing overseas. He had had great results with the products and was happy to recommend them. At the time he was an older man; but he was obviously fit and vital. To put it bluntly, he had the energy and drive I didn't!

You don't need a break down to have a breakthrough

While using detoxification products, one does not have to stop living and go through a health crisis. When I had been through multilple detoxes before, I had to take days or weekends off and suffer through the detox. It is important to find a product that not only allows you to continue on with your life, but also allows your body to truly heal.

You can apply these principles to any physical condition. For people with fibroid-myalgia, chronic fatigue,

Irritable Bowel Syndrome, chemical sensitivity and toxicity a good cleansing product will help. Ask your HealthSource Doctor or seek out a trusted health care provider that is versed in alternative healing methods. With their help, the process of detoxing is easy to begin.

Working with the experts

You will be asked to fill out a health appraisal questionnaire which will pinpoint which cleanse is right for you. Each of us has different issues that need to be addressed. Some of us have livers that function in a different phase of detoxification. Remember that we are after optimum health, which will only help us to maintain our healthy weight.

Tips to Detoxifying

#1 Follow the guide as to which foods to increase and which foods to eliminate.

#2 Cut back or eliminate coffee and nicotine. For most of us, coffee is our drug of choice. It is recommended that you forego coffee while on your detox.

#3 Start slowly. Wean yourself. This will help to avoid headaches.

#4 Avoid alcohol. Alcohol taxes the liver. You will need your liver operating at its highest level to process the toxins out of your body.

#5 Pump yourself with enthusiasm. Listen to your relaxation sessions. Spend time with your BRD (described in this book) staying positive will go a long way in building the attitude of a healthy person.

#6 Eliminate processed meats. Most people will elect to give up all meat during their cleanse. However, there is hope if you'd like to stay a carnivore. Your meat choices will be fresh or even frozen chicken, turkey, wild game, lamb and fresh or water packed fish. Wild game is easy to come by here in Maine. And, with the growth of high end natural food stores across the country, organic meats are available almost everywhere.

Watch out for the Road Blocks

One of my pitfalls and roadblocks to help was not knowing the complexity of the human liver. As I mentioned, I did not know that the liver would "shut down" if it was starved of protein, and in a time frame of less than three days. It is important that you select a product that never starves the body of protein, and that binds the free radicals as they leave the body. Your HealthSource Doctor will have recommendations for a complete program.

The Importance of the Four R's

R # 1 = REMOVE: When we remove toxins from the body, we start the path to complete healing. If something is there that is bothering the body, simply adding vitamins or nutrients will not stop the damage. We must also remove foods that someone may be allergic to.

When I was younger, people having food allergies was almost unheard of. Now, however, for whatever reason, most of us know people who are allergic to a host of things. With a moderate elimination diet, we can give the body a rest. Then later in the cycle add foods that may have been causing an allergic reaction. There will be trial and error during this process. What has always amazed me in clinical practice is how many people are allergic to their own favorite foods, hence why they are so ill.

R #2 – REPLACE: We must now replace what was lacking in our digestive tract, what was not allowing our bodies to properly digest our food. Most people that have indigestion after a meal, or feel full for an extended period, have bloating or gas or persistent diarrhea after eating will need some help replacing their bodies own digestive enzymes. As you may suspect , fiber is often lacking and needs to be present for optimal detoxification to take place.

R #3 REINOCULATION: After all the hard work of detoxification, the body and bowels will be extra clean, and need some help with re-inoculation of the good flora. Most of us are used to hearing people needing good flora after a bout of antibiotics. In my opinion, that's why most of us get in trouble in the first place. Two most commonly used (and studied) flora replacements are acidophilus and bifidus.

Both of these are present in young healthy people and when studied show a decrease as we age. I will put out the question whether they decrease due to drug use in the aging population. Sadly, a host of issues accompanies the lack of "good" flora, but for the purpose of this book, weight gain is noted. Live cultures are best, and will spur the body on toward proper function.

R #4 REPAIR: We must repair what has been damaged. We must heal the bowels and heal the liver. As we age and become more toxic, we often suffer from subtle but chronic nutritional insufficiencies, and food allergies--and if we are pushed too far, inflammatory bowel condition. The body must be given proper nutrients if it is to repair damage done. To be fully healthy and become a body that is naturally thin, detoxification must be complete and total. A halfway measure will only ensure that the cycle of illness and weight gain continues.

The complexities of proper detox are immense. No longer will the simple carrot juice and fasting suffice. It is tragic that for the lack of a few simple nutrients and protein, people are damaging what they are trying to heal.

Increasing Water Is The First Step

My own simple advice is to start detoxifying now. Put down the book and have a large glass of water. It is a simple fact that is often overlooked that most of us are dehydrated to one degree or another. This simple step will be a stepping stone to the more complex steps in the detox program.

Eliminate junk food. I found that having healthy snacks around would not only keep me happy, but work to keep me healthy as well. I suggest raw almonds, cashews, walnuts, sunflower, and pumpkin seeds. These would keep me from having junk and give me the energy that I desired.

Remember that you will have good days and bad days on the cleanse. If you find you are tired or sickly, look at what you are taking for detoxification. You may need to back off of your supplements. If you choose to detoxify without the benefit of a health professional, you may run the risk of improper detoxification, which will not only take longer but my require additional help with the repair process. All of us are toxic, but some more toxic than others. There is no need to do this alone. Two heads are always better than one; and your HealthSource doctor is there to help you.

Focus on the healthy life you are gaining, not on what you are giving up. You can look forward to being healthier and more vibrant. You will be well on your way to being the fit person of your dreams. Look at all the healthy things you CAN eat. Most people will elect a one month detox program. However, I have had patients who were extremely toxic or chemically compromised elect to stay on a program for up to six months. If that sounds long, remember that these people have never felt better in their lives--once their bodies were detoxed.

Success Is Up To You!

The rest is up to you. I am glad you have chosen me to help you on this journey, to be the guide I never had. It was chilling for me to have a doctor refuse to look me in the eyes, afraid they might have to talk to me about cancer. To then have a laundry list of liver diseases presented to me and then have to wait while they were eliminated by trial and error was a nightmare. I was then sent home with a liver that was not functional and given no options. It was time for me to take action.

I have options for you and they are all great. There is a better, stronger, younger healthier you! There really is! Every day you are beaten down with chemicals, airborne pollutants, overuse of drugs and bad foods. It is time for you to take control and commit to building a healthier, more vibrant you.

On this journey please know that you are not alone. Let this chapter be your guide as you look toward a horizon of health and vitality. You have the tools. Now let's build the new you!

> *"In minds crammed with thoughts, organs clogged with toxins, and bodies stiffened with neglect, there is just no space for anything else."*
> **~Alison Rose Levy, "An Ancient Cure for Modern Life," Yoga Journal, Jan/Feb 2002**

CHAPTER FOUR

FEEDING THE BODY -- BODY CHEMISTRY
BY AMANDA BORRE, DC

Feeding the Body-Body Chemistry
By Dr. Amanda Borré

When the subject of carbohydrates is brought up, a variety of opinions surface. I discovered through personal investigation that information on carbohydrates is available in copious amounts--some accurate, some not so. Some materials out there tout that eating carbohydrates is bad period. Entire books are written about how your body must have large amounts of carbohydrates to be healthy. It is really important that before making a decision on how carbohydrates fit into your life, you know the facts.

I have personally struggled with my weight my entire life. I was the only third grader with documented photos of my saddlebags! I have memories from childhood of rounding the corner in school or at the pool in the summertime to hear some rude teenager making fun of my size. Childhood obesity is no laughing matter. Being overweight and putting your health in jeopardy is funny to no one.

My goal in writing this chapter and contributing to this amazing book is to help others by sharing the knowledge I have gained through hundreds of hours of research. I hope that my saddlebags can lead to your success. Discover how carbohydrates are converted to sugar and released into the bloodstream and how this process affects your weight and your health. Continue reading to learn how you can adjust your carbohydrate intake to convert your body into a fat-burning machine!

A carbohydrate is named such because it is a glucose that is made of a carbon and water. The chemical make up of

CHAPTER 4 | FEEDING THE BODY -- BODY CHEMISTRY

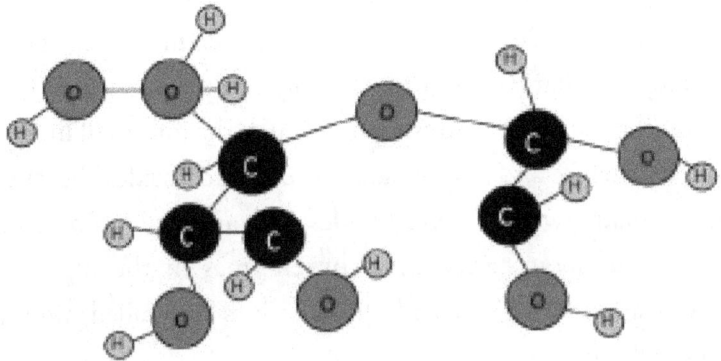

a food made from a carbohydrate, more commonly known as "carb," is 8 carbon molecules, 12 hydrogen molecules, and 8 oxygen molecules. It looks like the image above[1]:

Glucose is a "simple sugar" which means this is the basic structure. Foods containing glucose have a sweet taste on our tongue. Glucose plus fructose is called sucrose. It is found in fruits, vegetables, and table sugar. (Are you surprised to hear that the same chemical structure that is in a fruit is in table sugar? Read on for more surprises and how this can work FOR your weight loss-not against it!)

What is Lactose?

Lactose is glucose plus galactose. You have probably heard of someone being "lactose intolerant." Lactose is the sugar found in milk and milk products like ice cream and cheese. Usually the digestive process of this chemical does not work in a lactose intolerant body. Products are available to help break down those foods. All of these have the same chemical make up as glucose but with the atoms arranged differently.

Glucose, fructose and galactose all fall into the category of "monosaccharides" and are the only carbohydrates that can be absorbed into the bloodstream through the intestinal lining. Lactose, sucrose and maltose are called "disaccharides" because they contain two monosaccharides and are easily converted to their monosaccharide bases by enzymes in the digestive tract. Monosaccharides and disaccharides are called simple carbohydrates.

What is a Complex Carbohydrate?

A complex carbohydrate is made up of chains of glucose molecules. Most people know them as starches. Wheat, corn, rice, and potatoes are examples of a complex carbohydrate.

When you eat carbohydrates, the simplest form of digestion begins in your mouth. Large bites are chewed into smaller pieces. Remember when your mom said to chew every bite 100 times? It might have been overkill, but chewing properly is important in the digestive process. It starts it out on the right foot or, rather, tooth! Not only do your teeth do the work, but also your salivary glands produce an enzyme called salivary amylase.

What does Amylase Do?

This enzyme coats the tiny food pieces and essentially dissolves them into liquid form. This delightful concoction travels down your esophagus and into the stomach. In your stomach, digestive acids continue the breaking down of your food. From the stomach, the food travels to your intestines.

In your intestines these carbohydrates are broken into their smallest form such as glucose. The cells of the intestine (the intestinal epithelium) will then move the glucose across themselves and to their basal or, opposite, side. The basal side of the intestinal epithelium contains blood vessels, through which glucose can get into our bloodstream.

Glucose can now be taken to all of our cells. The body stores carbs as glycogen in your liver and in your muscle tissues.

What is the Process of Glycolyis?

The digestive system (the pancreas) also releases hormones such as insulin to get our cells to take up glucose even faster. When it needs energy, after depleting its stored supply of ATP (adenosine triphosphate), the body initiates glycolysis. Glycolysis is the process of converting carbs and sugar into ATP and ultimately energy. Specifically, a set of chemical reactions on glucose creates ATP, and a phosphate bond in ATP powers most of the machinery in any human cell.

When you eat a simple sugar, the digestion occurs very quickly because each of these processes does not have to be as long to break it down. This means your body can and will burn through these foods quicker.

What's So Important About Insulin?

The body is a wonderful machine and is able to maintain balance in your digestive system. When you have burned through the food you have eaten, your pancreas will need to produce insulin to keep your blood sugar up. Without it, you would experience low blood sugar that would lead to dizziness, lethargy, nausea, or a myriad of other health symptoms.

This system is a beautiful way to maintain balance after eating a simple sugar, but when you ask your body to perform this way frequently and/or over a long period of time, the excess work mandatory of the pancreas and the excess insulin production can be harmful to your body.

Insulin is very important to the way our body uses the glucose in our foods. The functions of insulin include enabling glucose to be transported across the cell membranes, converting glucose into glycogen for storage in the liver and muscles, preventing protein breakdown for energy, and to help excess glucose be converted into fat.

According to the Encyclopedia Britannica[2]:

Insulin is a simple protein in which two polypeptide chains of amino acids are joined by disulfide linkages. Insulin helps transfer glucose into cells so that they can oxidize the glucose to produce energy for the body. In adipose (fat) tissue, insulin facilitates the storage of glucose and its conversion to fatty acids. Insulin also slows the breakdown of fatty acids. In muscle it promotes the uptake of amino acids for making proteins. In the liver it helps convert glucose into glycogen (the storage carbohydrate of animals) and it decreases gluconeogenesis (the formation of glucose from non-carbohydrate sources). The action of insulin is opposed by glucagon, another pancreatic hormone, and by epinephrine.[3]

How Important Is Quantity?

This shows us how important it is to eat the right amount of the right types of carbohydrates for not only successful weight management, but also in order to control our moods and temperament. If we are only supplying our bodies with brief spurts of energy to use, our systems can be overworked, improperly supplied, and make for just a cranky day overall.

Exactly how do we manage the right balance? Fructose and galactose do not immediately raise blood glucose levels, since they are first sent to the liver to be converted into glucose. Fiber is not digested by our gastrointestinal system, so it passes through, aiding digestion and contributing to feelings of fullness. Foods containing fiber often raise blood sugar more slowly than those without it. Using the proper amounts of simple sugars and complex carbohydrates, dairy, proteins, fiber and fats, we can keep our blood sugar steady, put less stress on our body systems, and achieve weight loss success!

How do we even know about the existence of sugar?

Actually, it dates back to the days of Christopher Columbus and the Spanish Conquistadors. They are credited for first encountering sugar cane. The Spanish first brought it back to Europe for examination and research. It quickly found a home in a popular new alcoholic drink--rum! Years later it began to be used for a food supply as well.

Throughout history, food supply has been viewed as a status symbol. The wealthy had plenty of food and showed their status by overeating and carrying overweight physiques. The poor were slight of build and willowy in size. Foods such as sugar cane and its derivatives crept onto tables worldwide and became a staple in every household instead of a rare treat for the elite. Over time obesity and overuse of simple sugars have become an epidemic.

What's the Good Part?

Now that you know how carbohydrates are converted to sugar and released into your bloodstream, you can use this information to educate and motivate yourself on how to adjust carbohydrate intake to convert your body into a fat burning machine!

The first step is to identify what exactly you are eating. Any processed foods will generally be found in the inner isles of your grocery store. They will be packaged and the outside of the package will have nutritional information. When you look at the label, there is a category under carbohydrates termed sugars. These are the simple sugars we have been discussing. Reading these labels will help you with processed, packaged foods. These should be consumed in a very limited quantity.

A better choice would be a fresh, all natural food. Vegetables and fruits contain many vitamins, minerals, and phytochemicals (plant chemicals) that are beneficial to good health. They are low in calories, and are a good choice for a snack.

As a matter of fact, many vegetables and fruits contain a good amount of fiber and more fructose than glucose. Examples of fruits that do not raise blood sugar quickly are fresh cherries, plums, pears, and apples. Nuts, especially almonds, are high in protein and give you a boost in energy.

What about Bread?

When you are choosing any type of bread product, look for whole grains. When you vary your choices, choose wisely, and keep carbohydrate intake low, you will no doubt turn your body into a lean, mean, fat burning machine. A great, well balanced diet also has the fantastic side effect of providing various textures, flavors, and feelings in our mouths. This phenomenon is actually known as *mouth feel*.

These aspects of food provide much satisfaction. The assortment of crunchy, chewy, fruity, creamy, etc. in our eating plan keeps eating a satisfying task instead of a battle. You do not need high carbohydrate foods to feel satiated, or full.

For some people, certain recipes or foods have a comforting effect. You might even have a cookbook of family secret recipes that you like to make from time to time. By making healthy substitutions and decreasing the carbohydrate content, you can "have your cake and eat it, too"! Did you know that cream has less carbohydrates than milk?

One great tip is to always keep quick, high protein, low carb snacks easily accessible at your house, in your car, and at work. It is much easier to make healthy decisions when you have the time, and use these "cheater options" when you do not have the time. HealthSource Chiropractic and Progressive

Rehabilitation Clinics are located all over the United States. Their clinics feature a wonderful array of bars, wafers, shakes and snacks perfect for those on the go.

Do You Have A Plan?

Another crucial key is preplanning meals. One day per week, sit down and plan your meals for the entire week. Shop for fresh ingredients and prepare as much of your plan as possible. This will allow you to tally your carbohydrate intake and adjust as necessary. It is a great time saver and reduces mid-week stress.

If you are planning a higher carbohydrate splurge, it is best to have it pre or post workout to give your body that extra boost when it is needed instead of when you are planting on the couch for some lazy time.

Although carbohydrates are not recommended in high amounts, they are a necessary part of a healthy diet. Carbohydrates are the only fuel source for many vital organs, including the brain, central nervous system and kidneys. If you cut out too many carbohydrates, your body will go into ketosis.

Dorland's Medical Dictionary defines ketosis as: "ketosis (ke-to´sis) abnormally elevated concentration of ketone bodies in the body tissues and fluids when fatty acids are incompletely metabolized, a complication of diabetes mellitus, starvation, and alcoholism."[4]

Therefore, by cutting too many carohydrates from your diet, you essentially are mocking starvation from a chemical standpoint. This can cause headaches, thirst, bad breath, a metallic taste in your mouth, weakness, dizziness, nausea or a stomach ache, or difficulty sleeping. If you have consumed a large amount of carbohydrates on a regular basis, you may mildly experience some of these symptoms for a short while after reducing your regular carb intake.

If you experience these symptoms more than a few days, you may need to increase your carbohydrate intake slightly. If they are severe, or persistent, you should contact your doctor.

The long term effects of a no- or very low- carbohydrate diet have not been studied extensively, and no valid scientific studies are available on this. There are theories about the alternatives chosen in these types of diets. When you restrict carbohydrates, you have to choose wisely from all the other food groups.

Many who have designed versions of the low- or no-carb plans have steered followers into choosing from only one or two food groups such as protein and fats. This can be a recipe for disaster leading to heart disease and/or stroke.

Some trainers will boast protein as the only nutrient necessary to build muscle. This is simply untrue. The entire cast of nutrients is required for the process of muscle building. Only through a balanced diet with sufficient carbohydrate intake can the body reach its fullest muscle building potential.

When you keep your carbohydrate intake at a lean, reasonable level, your blood sugar will be held more constant, the amount of hormones released into your body is regulated, and you will experience a huge difference in the way you feel. Not only can the information included in this chapter be used for weight loss, but it can be utilized for elevation in mood, decrease in insomnia, lowered cholesterol, and improved health overall.

Today I am a healthy weight. It is not because I have grown into some super metabolism. I fight every day. Using these tips and the knowledge I have just shared helps me win, on a daily basis, the fight. You too can have success by adjusting your carbohydrate intake to convert your body into a fat-burning machine!

> *"Nothing will benefit human health and increase the chances for survival of life on Earth as much as the evolution to a vegetarian diet."*
> **Albert Einstein (1879 - 1955)**

References:
1. 2008 How Stuff Works
2. Yale Guide to Children's Nutrition
3. Encyclopedia Brittanica
4. Dorland's Medical Dictionary

CHAPTER FIVE

**Dispelling the Protein Myth
by Frank Dachtler, DC**

Dispelling the Protein Myth
by Frank Dachtler, DC

We have all likely heard the term protein and acknowledge that it is part of our diet. It's packed into a can of tuna, a chicken breast, and dairy products. Body builders live on it--and can eat an entire side of beef at a sitting... right? There are countless numbers of diet plans that emphasize the intake of protein; and in some cases NOTHING BUT this "miracle" nutrient. It even has its own line in the nutritional information window on food products. What exactly is protein? More importantly, "Why Is Protein Important to You?"

Before we discuss the absolute essential role that protein plays in our lives, let us address the euphemistic "elephant in the room," the myths about protein. One of the most common myths is that protein can be detrimental to your health as well as helpful. I have spoken on this topic to many of my patients over the years; some in consultation and many others in a lecture type setting. Inevitably, someone will explain to me their understanding of protein and its ill effects on the body--primarily the heart, colon and kidneys. Another common myth is one that deals with what the proper amount of protein the average person should consume daily. Thirdly, is that all proteins are the same regardless of their source. My favorite myth is that consuming protein makes you fat.

In this chapter we will discuss these myths in detail; but I encourage you to research this topic for yourself as well. As you begin to investigate the Protein Myth further, apply your past experiences, observations, and current knowledge base to this topic and I am confident you will arrive at the same conclusions that modern science and I have come to.

CHAPTER 5 | DISPELLING THE PROTEIN MYTH

What is Protein?

Protein is involved primarily as the building blocks of the human body. It makes up the mass of our body's enzymes, some hormones, hair, skin, cells of the internal organs, muscles, and brain tissue. Essentially, everything in your body that is not bone or fat is likely a result of protein intake. A protein is made up of much smaller molecules called amino acids that function as the actual compounds utilized by the body for growth. As we eat our meals, the protein that is contained in that food is broken down in the body. The result is amino acids. There are twenty different types of amino acids. Eight of these are called **essential amino acids**. Essential amino acids are ones that the body cannot manufacture on its own. They must be supplied in our food. Keep in mind, all amino acids are necessary for proper protein synthesis and thus normal body function. Deficiencies of one or more amino acids can have a wide range of harmful effects upon your health such as hair loss, dermatitis, weakness, fainting, fatigue, cold intolerance, headaches, anemia, elevated cholesterol, delayed healing, cardiac disorders, muscle cramping and abdominal pain to name just a few.

Having a diet rich in the proper amino acids not only helps build a strong, healthy system, but also increases your metabolism and thus helps your body burn fat. Fortunately, our body builds a "pool" or backup supply of these amino acids so that the many different proteins that the body needs can be produced at a moment's notice. Our job is to provide our body with those amino acids through proper diet and sufficient protein intake.

The closest thing to a health hazard resulting from protein intake deal with the immune system and allergies. Beyond that, there is very little evidence that protein leads to chronic disease. Protein was once thought to increase the risk of cardiovascular disease--primarily due to the fact that many protein source are also high in fat and low in carbohydrates. Recent studies have been performed where large amounts of protein, primarily from vegetable sources, actually reduced the risk of heart disease by 30% (*Halton TL, Willett WC, Liu S, et al. Low-carbohydrate-diet score and the risk of coronary heart disease in women. N Engl J Med. 2006; 355:1991–2002.*) Similar studies by Halton also suggest that diets high in fat and protein from vegetable sources significantly reduced the risk of type II diabetes.

There is no evidence showing any link between protein intake and cancer or colon disease. There is, however, a significant connection between processed meats and the risk of colon cancer. This has nothing to do though with the protein but rather the chemicals used in the preparation of certain food sources. There is evidence to suggest that diets high in red meat will tend to be deficient in fiber and therefore drastically affect colon health.

Does too much protein cause kidney issues?

The reality is that there are no studies showing a correlation between high protein diets and kidney problems in people with healthy kidneys. There are a few, however, that indicate people with existing kidney disease or diabetes may have some concern. Even in those studies, it took above normal protein intake to cause even the slightest changes in kidney function. If you are being treated for kidney disease or diabetes, you should always consult with your doctor first before making any extreme changes in your diet.

There are studies that show that protein deficiencies can actually cause kidney disease, though. One in particular, performed by Wojciech Swat, Ph.D, indicates that the lack of certain proteins can deactivate a specific hormone necessary for urine expulsion. This condition, which is known as functional obstruction, impairs the ureter's ability to pump urine from the kidney to the bladder. So it is unlikely that a diet high in protein will actually cause damage to the kidneys. The benefits of a balanced diet, with a sufficient amount of protein will far outweigh the negatives.

There has been some definite controversy over how much protein is enough. For years, bodybuilders and athletes have understood the importance of protein in their diets to maximize growth and recovery. Protein contains only 4 kcals per gram as opposed to the 9 kcals per gram contained in fat. Unlike fat and carbohydrates, excessive amounts of protein are not readily stored in the body for energy.

What does that mean? Proteins don't tend to make you fat! Protein speeds up the metabolism and contributes greatly to the increase of muscle growth. Increased muscle growth further turns you into a fat burning machine. Muscle burns away fat stores when at rest. So even when you're done exercising your muscles are trying to recover by moving the amino acids in and utilizing fat to do it.

So, again, what is enough protein? Typically, about .8 grams per pound of body weight. For example, a 160 lb. person will typically need about 128 grams of protein each day. Although this is commonly accepted as the rule of the day, the reality is that this number is just an estimate. Protein needs increase and decrease based on a number of variables including exercise type and length, weight gain or loss goals, male or female and illness.

When weight loss is the intention, calorie intake usually drops because you will (or at least should) drastically reduce fat and carbohydrate intake to shed the body fat. Much like a professional athlete, you may need upwards of 1.5 grams of protein per pound, to keep your body from burning muscle tissue for energy. Also, the more intense your exercise schedule and the amount of stress you have in your life affect the amount of protein you need.

Who is likely to have protein deficiency?

One thing is for sure, people living in the US are very unlikely to suffer from protein deficiency. Sources of protein are readily available and in most cases affordable. To become protein deficient you would either have to be on a starvation diet, have a metabolic disorder which would need to be treated medically, or you would have to eat nothing but low-protein, high-carb junk foods and certain fruits. If any of these are the case though, protein deficiency is going to be the least of your worries.

Are all proteins the same?

Not all protein sources and types are the same. As we mentioned earlier, they are made up of amino acids and there are twenty different types. That makes for quite an extensive list but we can categorize them into two main groups--Complete Proteins and Incomplete Proteins.

<u>Complete proteins</u> are those that include most of the essential amino acids the body needs in their composition. They are typically derived from animals and are one of the few reliable source of vitamin B12. The downside, though, is that they usually do not contain sufficient amounts of fiber and often contain large amounts of saturated fat and cholesterol.

Common sources of complete proteins include red meat, pork, chicken, fish, dairy products, and eggs. Red meat, pork, processed meats (like hot dogs and bacon) and dairy products tend to contain the higher amounts of saturated fats. For example, a 12oz Porterhouse Steak--which sounds good and has enough meat to satisfy a 300 lb. offensive lineman--contains a whopping 75 grams of protein but also almost 90 grams of FAT, 35 of which are saturated fats.

A piece of fish like salmon or mackerel contains about the same amount of protein and fat but only a quarter of the amount of saturated fat. Three ounces of tuna (in water) or two cups of lentils will give you the same amount of protein as the 12 oz belly buster steak, but less than 2 grams of fat.

What are incomplete proteins?

Incomplete protein comes from fruits and vegetables. The name incomplete however is a bit of a misnomer. At one time, these foods were considered to be very low in one or more of the essential amino acids. It was theorized in a book by Frances Moore Lappe', *"Diet for a Small Planet" – 1971*, that foods like beans and rice for example, needed to be combined to form meals that contained complete proteins. This was later found to be completely false, and Lappé herself reversed her original theory.

The body will build up pools of amino acids when we eat proteins that can be drawn on later based upon the bodies needs. Fruits, vegetables, nuts, seeds, legumes, and grains all vary in their protein content and amino acid types but this is no different than the variations that also exist in meat and dairy sources. It is typically true, though, that the concentration of protein in a complete protein source is higher than that in an incomplete source. It is also possible that vitamin B12 will be lower in incomplete proteins and in some extreme cases, would need to be supplemented.

The good news for vegetarians, however, is that soybeans are one of the few sources of protein that will supply the most complete list of the amino acids which will give a little more flexibility when planning meals. As far as a protein source, many plants are abundant in protein. Lettuce, broccoli, cauliflower and spinach get anywhere from 34% to 49% of its calories from protein! Even celery can boast a 21% caloric value from protein. Beans and legumes can range anywhere from 25% to 55% depending on the type. Grains are 8% to 31%. Nuts and seeds are 8% to 21%. Fruits are the lowest at around 5-8%

on average. The advantage to obtaining the majority of your protein from these sources is that they are typically low in fat and high in fiber, and fiber is essential in helping our bodies balance blood sugar and in maintaining a healthy colon.

Another difference in proteins is the body's ability to digest them. Sources from egg whites, whey and fish will digest and reach the blood stream much quicker than the protein from sources like red meat, chicken, dairy, vegetables and whole eggs. The ideal time to consume the faster-digesting proteins is in the morning (to reverse the overnight fast); and before and after exercise, because the body needs immediate sources of protein to help prevent muscle breakdown and is more geared for protein intake into the cells. The slower-digesting proteins are just as healthy but more suited for moderate intake throughout the day and will assist in maintaining your body's metabolism and blood sugar levels indirectly.

Is it really possible to eat more and weigh less?

Based on the number of overweight and obese individuals in the United States--roughly two thirds of us--our first reaction would be no. The reality is that it is not necessarily the amount of food and thus caloric intake that causes us to become overweight. It is the type of foods we eat and when we eat them that are the biggest factors. Foods high in saturated fat, carbohydrates (in the form of processed sugars), and sodium will pack on the unwanted pounds while an equal amount of calories in the form of complex carbohydrates and protein can actually cause us to lose excess body fat!

What happens on a high protein diet?

When people eat lots of protein but few carbohydrates their metabolism changes into a state called *ketosis*. Ketosis means the body converts from burning carbs for fuel to burning its own fat. When fat is broken down, small bits of carbon called *ketones* are released into the bloodstream as energy sources. Ketosis, which also occurs in diabetes, tends to suppress appetite, causing people to eat less, and it also increases the body's elimination of fluids through urine, resulting in a loss of water weight

Note that the excess of anything--whether it is protein, carbohydrates or fat--will cause you to put on weight. If you require 2,200 calories a day to meet your requirements but still sit down in front of the TV and finish a bag of potato chips twenty minutes before you go to bed, the excess will be sent to the liver, converted to glucose and eventually make its way to fat stores. Protein seems to be a little less efficient at making body fat than dietary fat and carbohydrates, but please do not think that eating nothing but protein gives you a free pass on eating as much as you want. Protein is not completely exempt from being converted in the body into fat.

Conclusion.

So, don't be afraid of loading up on the protein. But keep in mind that this is only one small part of balanced and healthy lifestyle. Carbohydrates, fat, water and overall caloric intake should also be maintained. And of course, don't forget EXERCISE!! My hope is that you read these chapters with an open mind and take the time to sit down and develop a plan that is right for you. Then, act on that plan to become the healthy, happy person you were meant to be.

We lift ourselves by our thought, we climb upon our vision of ourselves. If you want to enlarge your life, you must first enlarge your thought of it and of yourself. Hold the ideal of yourself as you long to be, always, everywhere - your ideal of what you long to attain - the ideal of health, efficiency, success.

Orison Swett Marden (1850 - 1924)

CHAPTER SIX

Sugar Awareness
by Dr. Brandon Pettke

Sugar Awareness
Dr. Brandon Pettke

In this chapter, you will learn the truth about refined sugar, artificial sweeteners, and stimulants; find out why 75% of overweight people have a biological imbalance involving insulin; learn how sugar stimulates the overproduction of insulin, which promotes fat storage; and, most importantly, learn how to conquer your sugar cravings and get your body burning fat fast!

Some Amazing Sugar Stats!

We all know too much sugar is not good for us, but do we, as Americans, really eat that much sugar? When I started researching the facts, I couldn't believe what I was reading. The average American consumes an astonishing 2-3 pounds of sugar each week! Just think about eating a big paper sack full of sugar in a week's time. WOW! It makes me feel kind of sick just thinking about it! It's not surprising considering that highly refined sugars in the forms of sucrose (table sugar), dextrose (corn sugar), and high-fructose corn syrup are being processed into so many foods that we eat on a daily basis.

The average American eats an astounding 41.5 pounds of high fructose corn syrup per year.[1] In the last 20 years our country has increased it's table sugar consumption from 26 pounds to 135 pounds of sugar per person per year! Prior to the turn of this century (1887-1890), the average consumption was only 5 pounds per person per year.

Sit back and let those numbers sink in… that's A LOT of sugar!

In just a little over 100 years, we have DRASTICALLY

changed what we consume as Americans. The majority of change has been in the last 30 years, which just happens to correlate with the drastic rise in obesity and Type II diabetes. Hmmm… there seems to be a connection here, huh?

It is my hope the rest of this chapter will shed some light on this national problem and help you to understand *(without using too much scientific mumbo jumbo)* what is happening to your body and what you can do to drop the pounds dramatically.

Types of Sugars

There are several primary categories of sugar, which are categorized by their source. The most well-known sugar is sucrose, from which table sugar is derived. Sucrose comes from sugar beets or sugar cane. Fruit sugar is called fructose. Milk sugar is called lactose. Malt sugar is called maltose; and sugar from honey or sweet fruits is called glucose *(also called dextrose, corn sugar, or grape sugar)*.

Fructose is the sweetest sugar and lactose is the least sweet. To give you a perspective for sweetness, I will give each sugar an un-scientific "score". If I were to arbitrarily assign a "sweetness score" of 100 to fructose, sucrose would score a 58, glucose a 43, maltose a 19, and lactose a 9. The potency of sweetness of a particular sugar does not make it inherently bad, or good. I am simply giving you "scores" now, because I will be referencing them in later sections of this chapter.

The Most Consumed "Sugar"… It's Everywhere!

The number one source of calories for Americans is now High Fructose Corn Syrup (HFCS). It is the sweetener and sugar of choice for countless processed foods, soft drinks, and even some "health foods". It is everywhere and it is detrimental to our health and our waistlines--and we don't even realize it!

The number one source of HFCS for Americans is soft drinks. They account for more than one quarter of all drinks consumed in the United States. More than 15 billion--yes, that's BILLION--gallons were sold in the U.S. in the year 2000. Not only are soft drinks widely available everywhere, from fast food restaurants to video stores, they're now sold in 60 % of all public and private middle schools and high schools nationwide according to the National Soft Drink Association.[2]

It doesn't just stop with soft drinks. HFCS is everywhere. Start looking at the labels on all the processed, bottled and boxed foods in the middle aisles of your supermarket. The majority of these products have high fructose corn syrup in their ingredients list. Every thing from peanut butter to salad dressings to spaghetti sauces to canned fruit to boxed meals that just need chicken or hamburger added....I could list thousands of items, but I think you get the point. Simply start reading labels and stay clear of this stuff! It is only helping keep the pounds on and packing more fat on for extra measure! You will see and understand why a little later.

How HFCS Is Made?

According to Mark Sisson, a fitness and health expert, "HFCS is made by soaking corn and allowing it to separate. The sugar present in the cornstarch is processed (with the use of enzymes) to increase fructose content. Corn syrup is then added. The resulting HFCS contains some proportion of fructose to glucose depending on its intended use (typically 55:45 for soft drinks, 42:58 for many baked goods)."

Remember how much sweeter fructose is than sucrose (100:58)? Sisson goes on to explain, "HFCS isn't processed by the body in the same way as sucrose. Instead of setting off a hormonal chain of events and responses involving insulin and leptin, which helps us regulate food intake, HFCS skips over this process. The body doesn't recognize it in the same capacity.

Hence, HFCS doesn't "trip" the same switch to tell us we've had enough. So we keep eating more. HFCS's processing in the liver results in an insidious elevation of blood triglycerides, and it's more readily turned into fat storage." This, in turn, leads to a higher risk for obesity, insulin resistance (which we will speak on later), cardiovascular disease, some cancers, and Metabolic Syndrome.

"Health Foods" With HFCS

Generally speaking, the most common "health foods" that contain HFCS are fat-free or reduced fat products. If you take the fat out of a product it changes the taste of that product. Therefore, you have to add something else make it taste good or it will not sell. A cheap method to improve taste of these products is HFCS.

Here is a list of 6 commonly consumed "health foods" that are filled with High Fructose Corn Syrup that contribute to keeping your weight on.[3]:

- *Yoplait® Yogurt*
Oh yes, every variety of Yoplait contains HFCS!

- *Salad Dressings*
Most salad dressings contain HFCS, but "lite" and "reduced calorie" versions are brimming with it. Prior to the no-fat craze, salad dressings were typically made with cheap, poor-quality corn oil. Now they're made with cheap, poor-quality HFCS.

- ***"Smart" Ice Cream Sandwiches***

Many low-calorie ice cream treats are packed with upwards of 20 grams of this nutritionally deficient sweetener (HFCS).

- ***Special K®***

It's high time for most cereals to stop proclaiming health benefits. Made from grains, gums and sugars, which all increase fat deposits, there's nothing smart about cereal for breakfast--no matter how special it may be.

- ***Cereals with the Heart Healthy Claims***

Many breakfast cereals are loaded with HFCS and processed junk, but because they have a few grams of fiber or are low in fat, they are promoted as health foods.

- ***100 Calorie Snack Packs***

We're all in favor of portion control, but it's what's in the package that matters. You're much better off eating 100 calories of almonds or sugar snap peas than some processed cookie confection.

If HFCS Is So Bad, Then Why Is It Everywhere?

Here's the simple answer: The reason HFCS is so prevalent is because it is much cheaper to produce and manufacture than sugar (sucrose). It simply comes down to finances for food and beverage companies. However, just because it is more profitable for them to use HFCS doesn't mean that it is as healthy or healthier for you, no matter what the marketing gurus say! Ultimately, you have to take responsibility for your own weight and health. I hope after reading this chapter and book, you will take the steps necessary to do so.

Glycemic Index: What The Heck Is This?

The Glycemic Index (GI) is the comparable measure of how quickly foods and beverages will raise your blood sugar (glucose) levels. Eating pure glucose is given a ranking of 100 on the Glycemic Index. All other foods are compared in relation to this.

So a food with a Glycemic Index of 95 raises blood sugar almost as much as pure glucose, but a food with a Glycemic Index of 20 doesn't raise blood sugar much at all. It's important to keep in mind that the Glycemic Index does not take portion size into account.

The actual amount any food raises blood sugar has to do both with how glycemic it is and how much of it you eat. What is termed the Glycemic Load (GL) attempts to combine these concepts.

We will come back and reference Glycemic Index later on in the chapter. For now, here is a brief chart to give you an idea:

Beer	110
Glucose	100
Baked Potato	93
Rice Cakes	91
Pretzels	83
White Bread	70
Whole Wheat Bread	69
Cantaloupe	65
Corn	55
Banana	55
Stone Ground Whole Wheat Bread	53
Baked Beans	48
Lentils	30
Milk- Whole	22
Broccoli	10
Onions	10

Insulin: Too Much Of It, For Too Long Will Get You Fat & Keep You Fat

I am going to try and keep a complex scientific topic relatively simple. You gotta stay with me on this longer section. It's very important for you to understand this process if you want to lose weight. Okay? Here we go!

You have basically three types of foods you can eat: proteins, fats, and carbohydrates. Proteins and fats have very little effect on blood sugar level. Carbohydrates do affect blood sugar levels which, in turn, affect insulin levels.

There are different types of carbohydrates. But no matter what kind you eat, they are absorbed into the blood as sugar (glucose). This is true if you eat a bowl of broccoli or a bowl of table sugar. The difference between broccoli and table sugar is how quickly the glucose gets into the blood. The measure of how quickly this occurs is the Glycemic Index (see earlier in this chapter). The higher the number on the Glycemic Index, the faster glucose gets into the blood stream.

With broccoli, a rise in blood sugar levels occurs very slowly. The broccoli has to be absorbed and broken down. The digestible carbohydrate has to be broken away from the un-digestible fiber. This whole process will raise blood sugar levels very slowly, over about a 2 hour time frame.

With table sugar, blood sugar levels rise almost instantaneously. With a pretzel or saltine cracker, blood sugar levels don't take much longer than table sugar to rise. Try this experiment with either a pretzel or a saltine cracker: Put one in your mouth and start chewing. After about 8-10 seconds you will start to have a sweet taste in your mouth. This is because in your saliva is an enzyme called amylase, which starts breaking down these carbohydrates into sugars. Increased blood sugar levels lead the pancreas to secrete insulin. Insulin is the hormone that moves sugar (glucose) from the blood stream, into the cells Fig 1.

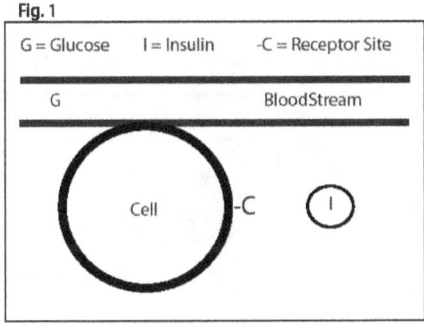

Fig. 1

Each cell in the body has what are called receptor sites on them. There can be receptor sites for many things like proteins, hormones (i.e. insulin), etc. In our scenario, think of the receptor sites and insulin like a deadbolt and a key. The deadbolt is the receptor site and insulin is the key. Once insulin connects to the receptor site on the cell--like a key unlocking a deadbolt-- insulin then opens up a channel connecting the cell to the bloodstream.

This allows glucose molecules to come into the cell. To give you a visual, think of a using the key to open the front door of your house. Once the door is open you (glucose) are allowed into the house (cell) Fig 2.

Once the glucose is in the cell, the glucose molecule will go through a chain of reactions and energy will be extracted from it. Each cell will then use that energy to do what it is supposed to do. If it is a kidney cell, it

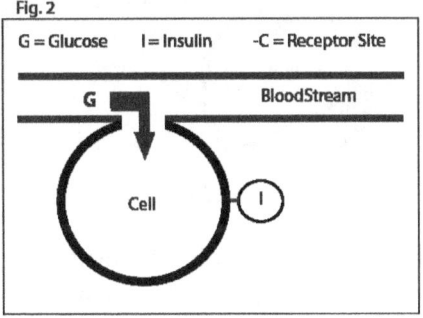

Fig. 2

will do kidney things. A liver cell will do liver things. A muscle cell will contract. However, if it is a FAT cell, it does not burn the glucose. The FAT cell converts glucose into fat because that's its job. FAT cells are storage units of energy; and FAT cells will keep the energy stored until needed.

When FAT cells convert glucose to fat, they pack fat up against the cell wall to make more room for other fat to be stored [Fig 3]. When blood sugar levels get low in between meals, *(and insulin is no longer connected to the receptor site of the fat cell)* our FAT cells are supposed to convert that fat into what are called Free Fatty Acids (FFA). Once fat is converted to FFA, it can 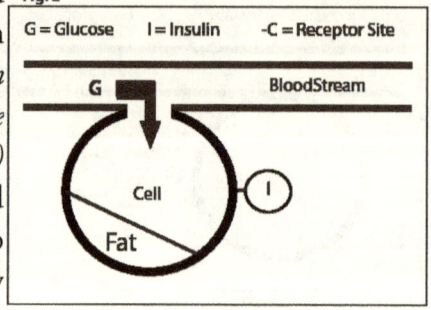 be moved back into the bloodstream as an energy molecule for other cells to utilize *(very similarly to how other cells would use glucose to perform functions)* [Fig 4]. This allows fat cells to not plump up, and keeps you thin.

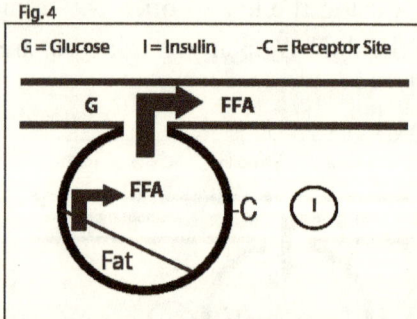 Herein lies the problem. If insulin is still connected to the receptor site, it will not allow the fat in a FAT cell to be converted to FFA. If it is not converted to FFA, it stays packed in the cell as fat and we can't utilize our own body fat. So the next time a big influx of sugar is in the blood stream, FAT cells take glucose inside the cell again, convert it into fat, and pack it on top of the fat that is already in the FAT cell [Fig 5]. If this process happens enough, you get larger and larger fat cells and gain unwanted weight.

Here's how this can happen. If we eat foods that are high on the Glycemic Index, like a baked potato for instance,

CHAPTER 6 | SUGAR AWARENESS

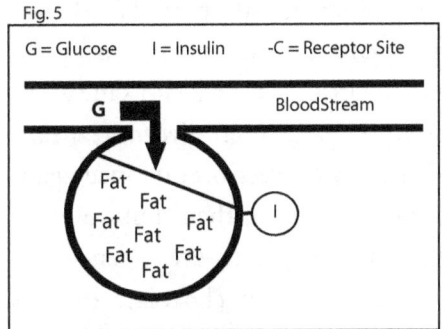

Fig. 5

this will produce a rapid influx of sugar into the blood stream. This will, in turn, produce a ton of insulin. The influx of insulin will then drop blood sugar levels fairly quickly; however, insulin is a long chain polypeptide hormone and it does not go away very quickly.

It has to be metabolized and its levels drop very slowly. This means that the blood stream no longer has much sugar in it but still has a lot of insulin. So the insulin is not allowing your FAT cells to convert stored fat into FFA to be used by other cells [Fig 6]. If these other cells don't have the readily available glucose or FFA that they need, you will feel tired and weak and then get a craving of "I need to eat or snack on something."

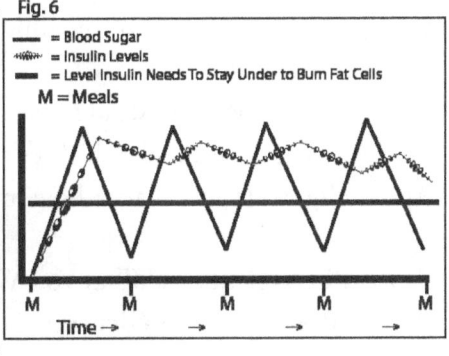

Fig. 6

Let me take you through a typical American's day: They eat breakfast at 7:30 am with a bowl of cereal, a banana, a strawberry yogurt (sweetened with HFCS), a glass of juice and a cup of coffee. Sounds pretty "healthy", huh? This is a high glycemic meal. The above mentioned process with blood sugar and insulin occurs [Fig 6]. At about 10 am they are feeling tired and have a craving for a snack. So they go and grab a donut someone has brought into the break room, and a cup of coffee.

This again is a high glycemic meal. The same blood

sugar spike and insulin routine occurs. At about 12:30 they are feeling tired and hungry again. So they go out and get a hamburger, French fries and a soft drink; or a sub sandwich, chips, and a sports drink--once again, high glycemic meals. The same blood sugar and insulin process occurs once again $^{Fig\ 6}$. At 3 pm they lay their head down on their desk for a 10 minute nap because they just can't keep their eyes open.

Maybe now they eat a couple of chocolate candies in their drawer or grab a soft drink or even a sugar-loaded "energy" drink--their choice. Same process occurs again with the insulin and blood sugar $^{Fig\ 6}$. Now when they get home they don't have any energy for their spouse or their kids. They sit down to eat dinner at 6:30 pm--maybe a big plate of spaghetti with some garlic toast and a sweet tea. Another high glycemic meal! 9:30 or 10 pm rolls around and you get a craving to get some ice cream, chips, or some popcorn. You guessed it! Another high glycemic meal.

Have I beat this dead horse enough? Practically no one can lose weight eating like this! It's physiologically impossible! And it almost doesn't matter how much you exercise!

Insulin Resistance: What You Will Get If You Do The Previous High Glycemic Scenario Too Long

I heard this analogy described one time for insulin resistance. It is very fitting and a very good mental image.

Let's say you moved into a house next to a railroad track. At first you notice the train engine going by because it is nice and loud. Eventually, over time, you get used to the train engine and you pay it no attention when it passes by. But, what happens when your friends come over for dinner and the train goes by? They almost jump out of their chairs because it is so loud. They ask, "How can you live here with all that noise?" You reply back, "What noise?" Because you've become accustomed to it, you don't even really notice it anymore.

This is basically what happens to receptor sites and insulin. If you keep blood sugars up high enough, for large amounts of the day, for a long enough time in your life, your receptor sites on your cells will start to ignore lower levels of insulin. The pancreas will then try to secrete more insulin ("get louder") to make the receptor sites accept ("hear") the insulin. If this process continues long enough in this trend, your pancreas will one day not be able to keep up and make the amount of insulin that is needed to get glucose in the cells. This will keep glucose in the blood stream. High levels of glucose in your blood stream are dangerous to your health, and can even be deadly.

When you get to this point, you now have insulin resistance. Your diagnosis for this condition is Type II Adult Onset Diabetes. Once you have diabetes, unless you drastically change your diet and start exercising, you will have to start taking insulin shots. Taking injected insulin manages the problem in the short term, but in the long term only continues this downward spiral. Have you ever known anyone that, assuming they make no real lifestyle changes, the longer they take insulin, the higher the dosage will climb to keep their blood sugar levels at a normal range?

If you are not a Type II diabetic already, you can take the necessary steps to keep this from occurring. For the most part, your health is a choice. So my question is: ***What choice will you make?***

But What If I Eat Foods With Artificial Sweeteners, That Don't Spike My Blood Sugar Levels Up? That Will Help Me Lose Weight, Right?

For the answer to this, let's turn to some recent research that has come out on the subject. I'll let you make the determination on this.

A study revealed that eating artificially sweetened foods and drinking artificially sweetened beverages might hinder your body's ability to estimate calorie intake, thus boosting your inclination to overindulge[4].

Study on Artificial Sweeteners

- The first group of rats were given two liquids, both of which contained natural high-calorie sweeteners
- The second group of rats were given two liquids, one that was sweetened with saccharin (Sweet 'N Low®)
- Both groups were given a sweet, high-calorie chocolate-flavored snack after 10 days into the study

Findings From the Study

- Rats that were given the artificially flavored liquids had a more difficult time differentiating their calorie intake and displayed the tendency to overeat
- The rats given artificially sweetened drinks were found to consume three times more calories than rats that didn't receive any sweeteners in their drinks

Researchers came to the conclusion that an inability to distinguish calorie intake was brought on by artificial sweeteners. On the other hand, the artificial sweetener industry viewed the results of the study as "inconclusive because of the fact that it was tested solely on animals". They also stated that "artificial sweeteners played an active part in weight loss and were a valuable tool for weight control". Another spokesperson for the artificial sweetener industry added that it "wasn't necessary to cut back on artificial sweeteners because the FDA previously approved them". I'm sure they have no financial motive in these statements since it is a multi billion dollar industry.

Can you sense my sarcasm?

Foods and beverages that contain no-calorie artificial sweeteners may be ruining your ability to control your food intake and body weight according to new research by psychologists at Purdue University's Ingestive Behavior Research Center[5].

In their study, rats that ate yogurt sweetened with glucose (a simple sugar), when compared to rats that ate yogurt sweetened with the zero-calorie artificial sweetener saccharin (Sweet 'N Low®): They found the rats who ate saccharin:

- Consumed more calories (and didn't make up for it by cutting back later)
- Gained more weight
- Put on more body fat

It's thought that consuming artificial sweeteners breaks the connection between a sweet sensation and a high-calorie food, thereby changing your body's ability to regulate intake. Researchers concluded that consuming foods sweetened with saccharin would lead to greater weight gain and body fat than eating the same foods sweetened with sugar. Although further research needs to be done, the researchers believe that consuming other artificial sweeteners such as aspartame (NutraSweet®, Equal®), sucralose (Splenda®), and acesulfame K (Sunnet® and Sweet One®) would have similar effects.

New research[6] suggests that the body is not so easily fooled by artificial sweeteners, and that sugar substitutes are no key to weight loss—perhaps helping to explain why, despite a plethora of low-calorie food and drink, Americans are heavier than ever.

In a series of experiments, scientists at Purdue University compared weight gain and eating habits in rats whose diets were supplemented with sweetened food containing either zero-calorie saccharin (NutraSweet®) or sugar. The report, published in Behavioral Neuroscience, presents some counterintuitive findings: Animals fed with artificially sweetened yogurt over a two-week period consumed more calories and gained more weight — mostly in the form of fat — than animals eating yogurt flavored with glucose, a natural, high-calorie sweetener.

This is a continuation of work the Purdue group began in 2004, when they reported that animals consuming saccharin-sweetened liquids and snacks tended to eat more than animals fed high-calorie, sweetened foods. The new study, say the scientists, offers stronger evidence that how we eat may depend on automatic, conditioned responses to food that are beyond our control.

Like Pavlov's dog trained to salivate at the sound of a bell, animals are similarly trained to anticipate lots of calories when they taste something sweet. In nature, sweet foods are usually loaded with calories. When an animal eats a saccharin-flavored food with no calories, however—disrupting the sweetness and calorie link—the animal tends to eat more and gain more weight, the new study shows.

The study was even able to document at the physiological level that animals given artificial sweeteners responded differently to their food than those eating high-calorie sweetened foods. The sugar-fed rats, for example, showed the expected uptick in core body temperature at mealtime, corresponding to their anticipation of a bolus of calories that they would need to start burning off — a sort of metabolic revving of the energy engines.

The saccharin-fed animals, on the other hand, showed no such rise in temperature. "The animals that had the artificial sweetener appear to have a different anticipatory response," says Susan Swithers, a professor of psychological sciences at Purdue University and a co-author of the study. "They don't anticipate as many calories arriving." The net result is a more sluggish metabolism that stores, rather than burns, incoming excess calories.

Swithers states, "It's still a bit of a mystery why they are overeating, but we definitely have evidence that the animals getting artificially sweetened yogurt end up eating more calories than the ones getting calorically sweetened yogurt."

Swithers says that separate studies on humans have already shown a similar effect. A University of Texas Health Science Center survey in 2005 found that people who drink diet soft drinks may actually gain weight. In that study, for every can of diet soda people consumed each day there was a 41% increased risk of being overweight.

Swither states, "Even though our findings were in rats, the research could lead to a better understanding of how the human body responds to food."

This emerging research could, and probably eventually will, fully explain why so many Americans feel like they never can get, and keep, the excess weight off while eating a diet of low-calorie artificially sweetened foods. Do you happen to fall into this category of dieters?

With that being said, have you ever noticed that most people who are diet soft drink drinkers are overweight? This is just something that I have observed personally over the years. Maybe now research is showing us why.

So What Should I Eat Then!?

You actually have many, many options. Let me give you a quick scenario of what you could eat as opposed to the high glycemic meals scenario mentioned earlier in this chapter:

At 7:30 am you eat a 3 egg omelet with chopped veggies and some low fat cheese covered with some salsa, an apple/peach or strawberries and a glass of milk. At 10 am you have a protein bar or apple (optional). At 12:30 you have a green leafy salad with veggies and grilled chicken breast with vinaigrette dressing and a glass of water with lemon. At 3 pm you have another protein bar or protein shake (optional) or a handful of roasted/raw nuts (optional).

At 6:30 pm you have a fillet of salmon with broccoli, grilled squash, and a glass of tea sweetened with stevia, xylitol, or agave nectar (or trade it out with a 4 oz. glass of red wine). During the whole day you have plenty of energy, you don't feel tired and weak, and you don't feel the need, or craving, to snack.

The reason this occurs is because all the above mentioned items are low on the Glycemic Index and Glycemic Load. When they are low on the GI and GL, it allows blood sugar levels to rise slowly. When blood sugar levels rise slowly, insulin levels will raise near the same rate and there will not be spikes in insulin [Fig 7].

The blood sugar will also fall more slowly (because there is not a large spike in insulin), and insulin will fall at about the same rate. What this means is that in between meals insulin will not be keeping your FAT cells from converting fat

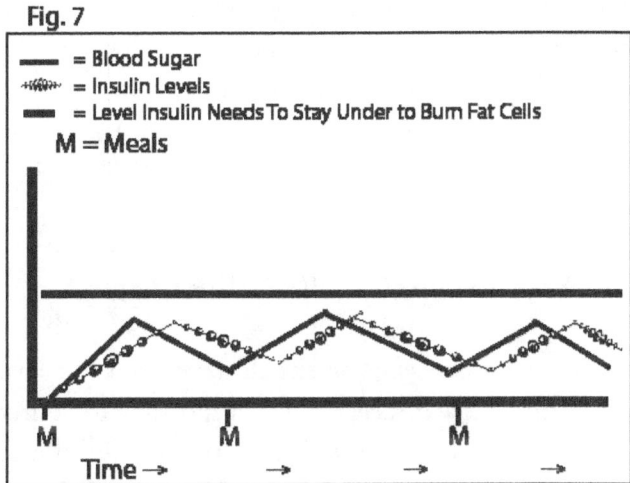

Fig. 7

to FFA and releasing it into the blood stream. This means you will be burning your fat in your FAT cells and you will lose weight! It's basic physiology and it works every time. Now you just have to apply your newly gained knowledge!

Here is a short list/guideline for you (high GI and GL foods):

Foods To Avoid:
1) *All Sweets*
2) *All Starches, Breads, Cereals (except cooked oatmeal), Crackers, Chips, Pasta, Potatoes (except yams), Rice*
3) *Only 2 Vegetables, Corn, Beets*
4) *Certain Fruits, Bananas, Cantaloupe, Honeydew, Kiwi, Mangos, Papaya, Watermelon, Dried Fruit (raisins, dates, etc.)- only exception is Apricots, All Fruit Juices*
5) *Alcohol, Beer, Sweet Wines*

Preferred Foods (low GI and GL foods):
1) *Fish*
2) *Meat (limit red meats 1-4X/month)*
3) *Dairy (limit to 3-5 servings per week)*

4) *Fruits (apple, orange, peach, plum, nectarine, all berries, pear and any others not listed above)*
5) *Nuts (almonds, walnuts, cashews, peanuts, etc.)*
6) *Vegetables, Vegetables--and oh yeah, more Vegetables (5+ servings of vegetables per day. Fresh or lightly steamed are preferable.)*

What Should I Take From This Chapter?

The main concept you should take from this chapter is to eat as many low glycemic foods as possible to your keep blood sugar levels low. This will, in turn, keep insulin levels low, which will allow your body to do two things: 1) Not pack on any more weight; and 2) burn the fat in the FAT molecules so you can get the trim body you want! If you stick with this principle, you WILL lose weight and keep it off!

*"Life can only be understood backwards;
but it must be lived forwards."*
Soren Kierkegaard (1813 - 1855)

References:
1. http://www.hfcsfacts.com/PerCapitaConsumption.html
2. Washington Post. February 27, 2001; Page HE10
3. http://www.marksdailyapple.com/sneaky-syrup/
4. International Journal of Obesity. July 2004; 28(7) Pages 933-935
5. Behavioral Neuroscience. February 2008, Vol. 22, No. 1, Pages 161-173
6. Behavioral Neuroscience. Swithers SE, Baker CR, Davidson TL. 2009 Aug;123(4): Pages 772-780

CHAPTER SEVEN

IMPORTANCE OF FIBER IN WEIGHT LOSS AND HEALTH
BY JESSI REZAC, MS

Fiber...Your Body's Best Friend
by Jessica Rezac, MS

FIBER....everybody's favorite five letter word! This chapter will answer some of your most common fiber questions such as: What is fiber? How do I know if I'm getting enough? Where can I get fiber? Is fiber really that important? Read on to find these answers and much more!

What is Fiber?

The term "fiber" was first used in the 1950s to describe the non-digestible part of plants. This means the part of the plant that goes through our digestive system without being broken down into usable pieces. However, fiber didn't become a household word until the 1970s when Dr. Burkitt and his team developed the "dietary fiber hypothesis." The dietary fiber hypothesis was a theory that states, "as fiber intake decreases, rates of heart disease & colon problems increase." They made this discovery after doing research in Africa and finding that common diseases in Western cultures--cardiovascular diseases such as heart attack and high blood pressure; metabolic disorders such as obesity and diabetes; intestinal problems such as constipation, diverticulitis, gallstones, appendicitis, hemorrhoids, polyps, and colon cancer; varicose veins and blood clots; deep vein thrombosis--were not common in Africa. The main difference between the cultures was their high intake of dietary fiber and low intake of refined carbohydrate. These diseases gradually increased in Western cultures as the use of new milling techniques that removed the fiber from the grain were used. Therefore, a lot of research has gone into determining which diseases fiber affects and how it affects it.

Fiber is so important for many processes that go on in our body. The one most people think of first is bowel function. Without adequate fiber, the gut and bowels don't function properly, slowing down the transport of waste out of the body, which can lead to constipation, bloating, toxicity, and diverticulitis. These issues can be very uncomfortable and can lead to more serious health problems.

Not only is fiber important for gut function, but other body systems as well. Fiber helps to keep blood sugar and cholesterol at normal levels. Fiber slows the absorption of food, thereby slowing the release of sugar into the blood stream and helping to maintain a normal blood sugar level. Eating fiber also offers good news for your heart! When people eat fiber rich foods frequently for breakfast, research shows they eat less fat and cholesterol the rest of the day than when they eat other types of breakfast. This is great for maintaining normal cholesterol levels and preventing heart disease.

Fiber and Weight Loss

I'm sure you're thinking, "It's great and all that fiber helps our intestines to function properly and our blood work to come back normal, but I want to lose weight. Can fiber help with that?" The answer is: YES IT CAN!

Fiber helps to stave off hunger, helps you to feel full faster and longer, makes it easier to reduce calories, and may reduce appetite. Let me explain how. As I've mentioned, fiber is the part of food that we can't digest, so it moves quickly through the intestinal tract. Fiber holds onto water, so it tends to be bulky in our stomach. This is how it fills us up and keeps us full for quite a while. As fiber leaves our stomach, enters the intestines and begins passing through, it takes with it the rest of our bodily waste. Fiber does this by holding onto water and scrubbing out the intestines as it passes. This keeps us regular, reduces belly bloat, and keeps weight down.

As an example, let me share Barb's story. Barb was one of my all star weight loss patients. She followed her weight loss plan exactly, and had already lost 70 pounds! Since she was feeling much better after losing so much weight, she began becoming more aware of her body and its functioning. She had always been very constipated--her whole life in fact. One simple recommendation I made was to add fiber to her breakfast. Her new breakfast consisted of old fashioned oats, steel cut oats, flaxseed, and blueberries. Just days after switching to this breakfast, she was suddenly very regular! It was as simple as adding a good sized amount of fiber to one meal! Here's the recipe Barb used:

My Secret Belly Slimming Breakfast

Bring 1 ¼ c water to a boil. Add ¼ c old fashioned oats and ¼ c steel cut oats, reduce heat to low and simmer for 10 minutes (or to desired consistency). Transfer oatmeal to bowl and add ½ T ground flaxseed, ½ T whole flaxseeds, and ¾ c blueberries. Enjoy! This meal has approximately 15 grams of fiber! That's half of your daily recommendation in one meal and a great way to start your day!

How Can I Get More Fiber in MY Diet?

Adding fiber to your diet is something you can start right away. It's simple and requires just a few changes to reach your daily goal of 25-30 grams or more. Here are some general guidelines to follow:

- increase intake of vegetables & fruits
- eat your veggies—aim for 5-10 or more servings/day (one serving equals ½ cup)
- choose fruit wisely—apples have 5g, Asian pear has 10, while 15 grapes have only 1
- add shredded veggies to soups, sandwiches, pizza, pasta, and other entrees
- increase intake of whole grains, while decreasing refined grain intake
- a whole grain bread or pasta is one where the first ingredient on the list is whole wheat flour, stone ground whole wheat flour, not enriched wheat flour
- eat whole rolled oats or steel cut oats daily, instead of instant oats
- choose cereals wisely--1 cup of Cheerios has 3 grams of fiber whereas 1 cup of Kashi Go Lean has 10 grams!
- supplement your diet with a protein shake that has fiber too
- add legumes and nuts to your diet
- add these to soups, chili's, and enchiladas
- substitute beans for meat in recipes

To reach your goal of at least 25 grams of fiber per day, you'll need to pay attention to food labels. Here is a sample

Nutrition Facts
Serving Size 1 cup 81g (81 g)

Amount Per Serving

Calories 307 — Calories from Fat 44

% Daily Value*

Total Fat 5g	8%
Saturated Fat 1g	4%
Trans Fat	
Cholesterol 0mg	0%
Sodium 5mg	0%
Total Carbohydrate 56g	19%
Dietary Fiber 8g	33%
Sugars 1g	
Protein 11g	

Vitamin A	0%	Vitamin C	0%
Calcium	4%	Iron	19%

*Percent Daily Values are based on a 2,000 calorie diet. Your daily values may be higher or lower depending on your calorie needs.

©www.NutritionData.com

Nutritional data and images courtesy of www.NutritionData.com.

label from a package of oatmeal.

Let me explain what to look for on this label in regards to fiber. At the top of the Nutrition Facts you can see that the serving size is 1 cup and that there are 307 calories in one serving. Under Total Carbohydrate, you can see Dietary Fiber is listed. Right next to Dietary Fiber it says 8g. This means that in one cup of oatmeal, you are consuming 8 grams of fiber. When you start monitoring your fiber intake, reading and understanding food labels is very important. It's the only way to know how much fiber you're actually getting from the foods you are choosing.

A great way to get started is to record how many grams of fiber you're currently eating, and then make adjustments (by following the suggestions previously listed) to your diet. But take it slow! If you go from 10 grams to 30 grams overnight, you may suffer from gas, bloating, or other digestive complaints. Gradually add a few grams each day until you've reached your goal. By upping your fiber intake to at least 25 grams per day, you'll start to notice changes right away. You'll feel full faster and stay satiated longer. You'll notice you have more regular bowel movements and your energy will increase.

Chapter 7 | Importance of Fiber in Weight Loss and Health

Your blood sugar will stay more regulated so your appetite will normalize, making it easier to stick to your weight loss plan. You will start to consume fewer calories without even noticing, therefore facilitating weight loss.

Popular doctor and author, Dr. Mehmet Oz suggests that women get 25 grams of fiber daily, while men need 35, by eating foods such as: steel-cut oatmeal, brown rice-pasta-bread, beans, 100% whole grains, psyllium husks, and chia (a Peruvian whole grain seed high in fiber, magnesium, calcium and omega-3 fatty acids).

Dr. Oz did an experiment on *The Oprah Winfrey Show* to see just how quickly and effectively a high fiber diet can start working. He took two truck drivers, Don and Wolfgang, and first measured just how slowly their guts were moving by having them swallow a pill with a tiny transmitter. The transmitter allowed the researchers to see how long it takes for them to process their food.

It took nearly a full day for Don to pass his pill and more than 42 hours for Wolfgang. Neither participant consumed a significant amount of fiber in their daily diet. Dr. Oz had the men load up on fiber for one week and swallow the transmitter again. Both significantly reduced their food transit times--Don cutting his time in half and Wolfgang cut his time down to just 12 hours. Dr. Oz says the positive effects of getting enough fiber happen "almost immediately." The fiber gets things moving through your system, including toxins, very quickly. "Bile, when it gets absorbed through the bowel, turns to cholesterol. So when you take a lot of fiber in your diet, you suck the bile out of you, and your cholesterol drops automatically."

Fiber also gets rid of sugar which helps diabetics. It's a

great tool if you want to lose weight because it makes you feel full," Dr. Oz comments. The average American gets just seven grams of fiber a day, but women need about 25 grams and men need about 35 grams per day. "That's somewhere between seven and nine helpings of fruits and vegetables," he says. However, if you radically increase your intake of fiber, you may feel gassy. "Your intestinal tract isn't ready for it," Dr. Oz says. The fiber in the bowel is permeated by all these bacteria, the bacteria eat the fiber, and they make gas. That's their waste product. So my recommendation is to build your fiber intake slowly into your diet. At the end of the day, you're probably going to have some gas, but it's a good sign because it means you're digesting food that's good for you (www.Oprah.com).

In conclusion, eating enough fiber is important for weight loss, bowel function, blood sugar regulation, and heart disease prevention. Fiber not only helps you to feel good on a daily basis, but helps to reduce your risk of chronic disease. So, take a look at your diet, and if need be, start slowly adding more fiber-rich foods to your menu!

"Getting my lifelong weight struggle under control has come from a process of treating myself as well as I treat others in every way."
Oprah Winfrey (1954 -)
O Magazine, August 2004

CHAPTER EIGHT

ENZYMES
THE MISSING LINK TO HEALTH
MASON ORTH, DC

The Role of Enzymes in Weight Loss
By Mason Orth, DC

An Introduction to Digestive Health

My interest in health was really borne out of my interest in science, especially in human biology. I was fascinated at the complexity of human physiology and our ability to affect our physiology based on what we put in our mouth. My interest grew as I became more involved in the health sciences and sports and related activities; and I really started turning towards human performance and the role of nutrition in human performance and how we could affect our biology and physiology based on what we ate.

The more I got into sports--and eventually weight lifting--I pursued the topic of health even more, especially as it related to nutrition and peak human performance. I began to experiment on myself with different diets and food combinations based on how you ate and what you ate and how you combine foods and time of day that you ate and tried to determine the best type of diet that worked to achieve peak energy levels as well as burning fat and maintaining muscle mass. So my studies of health continued to grow from there.

Enzymes came into the equation the more I understood about digestion and the importance of proper digestion, especially as it relates to nutrient availability in the body and how the body absorbs nutrients as well as gets rid of waste. The importance of enzymes became very clear to me. If you don't have proper enzymes, you ultimately don't have proper digestion, and that affects everything from your energy levels to detoxification to even weight loss and losing fat.

Proper digestion is absolutely essential for healthy GI function. We can define digestion as breaking complex molecules or food stuffs into more simple and smaller molecules or particles that are able to be absorbed by the body. The more efficient digestion is, the more efficient the whole GI system functions. It's more completely able to absorb nutrients from the foods we eat. Food that is not broken down ends up in the large intestine and the colon where we have a ton of bacteria that live there. Those bacteria use food that's not absorbed by our body for themselves.

The more food that makes it down there, the more the bacteria has to use for energy and growth. That can be a help or hindrance to us as far as our health goes based on the type of bacteria that's in our intestine. We know that approximately 70% or more of our immune system function is tied directly to the types of bacteria that live in our intestines. We have bacteria that are beneficial and we have bacteria that are harmful. The type of bacteria that we harbor in our intestines comes down to our diet. In that regard, digestion is very important, and I'll talk about that more later on in this chapter.

Proper digestion is important for your body to detox itself as well. The GI system ultimately is one of the main ways the body gets rid of waste and, based on digestion, that will determine how long it takes for waste to move along the large intestines. The longer that food takes to move, the more toxic it becomes and the more your body can absorb toxins from the waste. If digestion is incomplete, it can affect the transit time and how well your body will absorb toxins. So digestion is incredibly important for not just GI function but overall health as well.

Macronutrients and micronutrients--What are they and how do they impact your health?

If you are looking at a food label--which everyone should do--macronutrients are the primary things we see on the food label. They are fats, proteins and carbohydrates that make up the foods we eat. They are big molecules as opposed to the smaller molecules that are vitamins and minerals. This is what your body uses for energy and are the building blocks for every tissue in your body. Fats, proteins and carbohydrates are what enzymes break down so the body can use the energy, build and repair tissues and basically function. We will look more in depth at these fats, proteins and carbohydrates and how they're digested below.

Macronutrients supply energy. They are used to build everything from skin, muscles, organs, blood and enzymes. Carbohydrates, fats and proteins are the building blocks to all our cells. Fats make up cell membranes and all sorts of different tissues in our bodies. Proteins are used for basically every structure in our bodies, including enzymes. Too much of the wrong macronutrients, especially carbohydrates, tend to work against us and get stored as fat. Carbohydrates are the primary source of energy for most of the systems of the body; and one of the most important factors in whether or not you lose weight comes from what kind of carbohydrates you choose to eat.

There are two types of carbohydrates--starchy and fibrous. Starchy carbs are the sugar, pasta, bread, rolls, potatoes and things that are easily broken down by enzymes we have in our body. They are used as energy and stored as fat if we consume too many of them. Fibrous carbs are carbs that we do not have the enzymes to digest efficiently. These are the salads and vegetables. Their job is to provide bulk in the stool and help move the waste along the GI tract efficiently. It is important to have enough of these types of carbs in our diets.

Micronutrients are primarily composed of vitamins and minerals. Most absorption of vitamins and minerals occurs in the small and large intestines. These are not broken down by enzymes the way macronutrients are. They aren't made of proteins and carbohydrates. In most cases they are minerals. The role of micronutrients in digestion is essential. They are used in all the chemical pathways that use the nutrients and energy from our foods to build and repair tissue.

Chapter 8 | Enzymes -- The Missing Link to Health

Digestion--The Journey to Health

Digestion is a process that begins before you even take your first bite of food. This journey entails everything from your first smell of food to the elimination process. Think of a pickle or lemon or olive. Chances are, your salivary glands start working before you've even started chewing the actual food.

Once the food enters your mouth, the process gets underway fully. Chewing is the first step. Many of us don't realize the importance of taking our time and chewing our food completely. We hurry when we eat and this is terrible for digestion. Chewing breaks up our food and allows the enzymes from the saliva in our mouths to begin to do its work. The salivary enzymes come from our salivary glands and they begin the breakdown of starches or carbohydrates in our mouths. The more we chew the more the enzymes can work and digestion can begin.

Once we swallow, food ends up in our stomach. The stomach produces acid and that acid, in conjunction with stomach enzymes, breaks down the proteins that we eat. Proteins are the building blocks for every tissue in the body and also make up the backbone of most of our enzymes. The enzymes in the stomach break down the proteins into amino acids and those are absorbed by the body.

Upon leaving the stomach, the food enters the duodenum, the first part of the small intestine. There are enzymes at work here, too. The pancreas secretes enzymes and the gall bladder secretes bile. Fat, carbohydrates and proteins are further broken down here. This is the process of digestion. Once the food passes through the first part of the small intestine, digestion has occurred and the body is absorbing all the nutrients that enzymes have helped break down.

A healthy GI function helps or hinders weight loss. Improper digestion leads to slow and sluggish GI tract movement where waste can accumulate and sit for too long. If this happens, waste chemicals are absorbed back into the blood, which ultimately has to be cleaned by the liver. When the liver has to work harder to detoxify the body, it becomes much less efficient at turning fat into energy and this slows down weight loss. Fat isn't directly burned for energy as fat in most cases. Fat is taken from fat cells and brought to the liver to be turned into different types of energy through a process called: gluconeogenisis. If the liver is too busy and working too hard to detox the blood because of excess waste chemicals in the bowels, it can't efficiently change fat into useable energy. Ultimately weight loss slows or stops.

So you can see how proper GI function and proper elimination of wastes becomes very important to weight loss. You should be having a bowel movement daily. It's vital to have regular bowel movements for detoxification and to keep the liver functioning properly. It's the body's way of getting rid of unused food stuff, chemicals, dead blood cells and bacteria waste. You need to take steps to ensure that you become regular.

Proper Energy?

Proper energy is the body having the ability to efficiently extract the energy it needs from food. The only way it can do this is through proper digestion. As a practical application, think of it as having the energy to make it from breakfast to lunch without the need for a mid morning candy bar snack. It's making it from lunch to dinner without the mid-afternoon slump that sometimes hits us. People undergo these dips in energy because of the types of foods that they're consuming and the types of carbohydrates in those foods. Blood sugar levels are impacted based on what you eat and if you have dips and peaks in the blood sugar, your energy levels are going to be significantly affected.

If nutrients aren't available in the foods you're consuming, the body can't absorb the energy in the foods, and you won't have the energy you need to function properly. Nutrient availability only occurs when nutrients are liberated from the foods we eat. This occurs with proper digestion. (You're seeing how this all ties in together now, right?) Think of it as trying to get into an egg without breaking the shell. All the energy is stored inside the shell but we can't get to it. Enzymes are the method our bodies use to break the shell and access the nutrients. Without nutrient availability which occurs through proper digestion and through enzymes, the body doesn't have the chance to absorb nutrients. Without the enzymes, we don't extract the energy from food.

Optimal nutritional absorption is important because if we don't absorb the nutrients we're ingesting, our bodies will crave certain foods and energy will be low. And, in the case of trying to lose body fat, without proper energy, the body doesn't have the substances it needs to go about the process of burning fat. Not to mention the impact that improper digestion has on overall GI function, immune system function, detoxification and energy levels.

Enzymes--the Key to Proper Digestion

Enzymes are involved in all chemical reactions within the body. Enzymes are the molecules that break down other molecules into smaller parts. They move from place to place within the body breaking down other molecules but are not affected themselves. They are reusable. Think of worker ants going about their day chewing things up and then moving along.

There are a number of different classes of enzymes when it comes to digestion. In the macronutrient world there are lipases, which break down fats; proteases, which break down protein; and carbohydrateases, which break down carbohydrates, especially starchy carbs.

We have sites all over our bodies that produce enzymes, based on what is trying to occur. Enzymes are produced in glands such as the salivary glands in the mouth; glands in the lining of the stomach; and glands in the pancreas and proximal small intestine. As I mentioned earlier, the digestive enzymes in the mouth are primarily concerned with starting the digestive process and breaking down starchy carbohydrates. The enzymes in the stomach break down proteins into smaller, useable pieces. Enzymes in the small intestines and pancreas actually break down all three macronutrients.

Besides being produced naturally in the body, enzymes are available in the foods we eat. Certain foods contain high amounts of enzymes. These are the whole foods--foods that haven't been processed or heated in any way. Processing and heat destroys the enzymes available in whole natural foods. Most of the enzymes we could consume this way would come from raw fruits, vegetables, seeds, sprouted gains and legumes.

Enzyme Depletion

Eating the typical American diet is the primary culprit in enzyme depletion. We tend to eat highly processed foods that have been significantly broken down and come in a wrapper, box or from a restaurant. These foods don't have enzymes in them at all. Every enzyme that is going to be needed then has to come from our own bodies. We also tend to eat more quantities of foods than we need, and as we eat these large amounts of overly processed and overly cooked foods, our body has to pump massive amounts of enzymes from our glands to try and keep up. Believe it or not, these glands are just like a muscle. They can become fatigued. They can't keep up with the production. As the enzymes become depleted and the body can no longer keep up, the enzyme levels drop.

So what happens then? Since enzymes are the key to unlocking energy from food, incomplete break down of food occurs when there aren't enough enzymes being produced. That translates directly to low energy due to nutrient inavailability. The nutrients aren't available to be absorbed and that leads to improper digestion and absorption. We also see that the body's ability to absorb what nutrients there are is decreased because of improper digestion, directly related to the depletion of enzymes. And remember, as I told you earlier, then there is an overgrowth of bacteria which is not beneficial to our health at all. All this leads to slower elimination and an increased toxicity in the bowels.

As enzymes are depleted and digestion is incomplete, once again the liver must step up and take care of the waste that the bacteria in the intestines is creating. Just as we have waste when we eat, so does the bacteria and it's the liver's job to remove that toxic waste. As the liver becomes overworked, other functions--especially those related to weight loss--become secondary as the liver turns its focus to detoxifying the body instead of helping you lose weight.

Fat burning is affected when fat has to be converted to different chemicals that are used by the body for energy. That process is called Gluconeogenisis. What that means is creating glucose or blood sugar out of something other than blood sugar and the liver is the only place where this occurs efficiently. When the liver has to focus on detoxifying the blood to keep up with improper digestion, it's ability to convert fat into energy is secondary so the process of burning fat and losing weight slows down considerably.

Symptoms of Enzyme Depletion

- Overall fatigue--general body fatigue and low energy levels throughout most of the day.
- Constipation and diarrhea--sometimes constipated for several days followed by a day or two of diarrhea. No regularity to bowel movements at all.
- Weight gain--overworked liver can lead to weight gain for the reasons described above.
- Gas and Bloating--these are big signs of enzyme depletion. Gas is produced by the bacteria left by improper digestion.
- Heartburn--improper enzyme levels slow the emptying of food from the stomach and more acid than needed is produced which can cause heartburn.
- Lack of Weight Loss--if the scale is not moving and you are not losing body fat despite best efforts, you need to look to your digestion and elimination which ultimately leads you to enzyme levels. Check to ensure enzyme levels are adequate.

How can you treat low Enzyme Levels?

There are two ways to improve enzyme levels. There are endogenous enzymes, which are the enzymes your body produces. Then there are exogenous sources of enzymes. Those are the sources we touched on earlier--whole foods. Again, the foods to focus on are raw fruits and vegetables, seeds, grains, legumes. These are all great sources of enzymes and they bring other health benefits as well.

Another way to increase enzyme levels is through supplementation. They come in capsule form and are easily taken with a meal to aid in the digestive process. If you're not sure whether an enzyme supplement is a good one, consult your HealthSource doctor or call the manufacturer. Any enzyme you consume in supplement form should contain at a minimum amylase, lipase, and protease. Remember, those are your three macronutrients.

If your diet does consist mostly of cooked and processed foods, you really should be concerned about your enzyme levels. The average American only consumes less than one serving of fruits or vegetables daily, so my guess is that roughly nine out of ten Americans suffer from an enzyme deficiency.

Enzymes and Your Weight Loss Goals

Without enzymes life wouldn't exist. There is no simpler way to put it. The lack of enzymes is rampant in today's dietary habits, especially when you're trying to lose weight. Without enzymes your food is not properly digested. You do not absorb the nutrients and energy from food that your body so desperately needs. Losing weight--believe it or not--does require this energy. Your body requires this energy to undergo the chemical processes required to burn body fat. Without enzymes, you cannot get the nutrients from the foods you're eating. When this happens you do not properly eliminate wastes and your liver functioning backs up. Essentially that makes efficient weight loss impossible.

My recommendation to any of my patients to ensure that their GI system is working properly is to make sure they're getting proper amounts of enzymes through the foods they consume and through supplementation if necessary.

CHAPTER NINE

THE IMMUNE SYSTEMS
ROLE IN WEIGHT LOSS
MICHAEL J. PORTER

The Immune System's Role In Weight Loss
By Michael J. Porter

What Is Your Immune Response?

Have you gained weight even though you feel you eat right? When you exercise, instead of losing weight do you get hungrier? Have you stopped exercising out of frustration, then noticed yourself eating foods that make you feel better? If this scenario rings a bell, then this chapter is for you. What we will explore is how you may be sensitive to certain foods and how those foods may be affecting your immune system and compromising you metabolically.

The immune system is one of the most complex systems of the human body. Until recently, researchers, scientists and physicians have had little understanding of the structure and function of this system. It could be argued that one of the most important systems in the body is the immune system. If the immune system becomes compromised, then all of our bodily functions become compromised.

To build a strong immune system, first you need a little understanding on how it works. The basic components are the lymphatic system, white blood cells and their specialized groups, and the antibody mechanisms of the specialized organs. Scientists are gaining a better understanding of the immune system and what it takes to biochemically aid and support its function.

Chapter 9 | The Immune System And Weight Loss

Your immune system is a body-wide network of specialized cells and processes. One of these processes produces antibodies in response to a vast array of invading viruses, bacteria, chemicals, and other substances foreign to your body. Nature has endowed our immune system with very sophisticated methods to determine if a substance in the body is foreign or not. One method involves chemical markers called antigens, which are found on the cells of our bodies. Every life-form, from the simplest virus to humans themselves, has unique antigens that form part of its chemical fingerprint.

The immune system makes a specific antibody for each antigen, capable or recognizing and attacking only that one. As you become exposed to more and more antigens, you build a huge library of thousands of different antibodies, a lifelong immunologic memory encoded in proteins. With proper maintenance, it will protect you very well. In spite of all its complexity, the immune system boils down to two basic functions: recognizing "us" and killing "them."

What is Agglutination?

When an antibody encounters the antigen, a reaction called agglutination (literally gluing) occurs. For example, the antibody attaches to a viral antigen and makes it very sticky. When cells, viruses, parasites and bacteria are agglutinated, they stick together and clump up, which makes the job of disposal all the easier. This is a very powerful defense mechanism.

There is more to the agglutination story. All foods contain chemicals known as lectins. Lectins that are incompatible with one's blood type create negative reactions. For starters, they cause agglutination of the blood, meaning they make red blood cells "sticky" so they clump together. This results in a reduction in oxygen supply in the body and lowered immunity. Lectins can also interfere with protein digestion, block hormones, trigger immune reactions and impair absorption. This discovery that many lectins contained antigens that had A-like or B-like characteristics provided the scientific link between blood type and diet. "Rememarkably, however, it's implications would lie dormant, gathering dust for most of the 20th century – until a handful of scientists, doctors and nutritionists began to explore the connection," declares Dr. Peter J. D'Adamo, author of *Eat Right 4 Your Type*.

As I would often mention to clients, It doesn't matter whether you or I believe it. What matters is if your immune system believes it. While you're doing everything you have to do today, your immune system will be doing everything it has been programmed to do, easily, effortlessly and automatically. It is important to remember that the immune system has total autonomy. If it believes something is bad, our immune system exercises its authority to call forth all the body's energies to protect it. Once the immune cells have branded a food as an "invader," the food will trigger an immune response each time it is detected in the blood, regardless of how healthy it may seem. And once a food is tagged as a foreign invader, each subsequent exposure confirms this. This results in an incredible amount of resources being used to keep you healthy and eventually causing you to feel drained, tired and wore out. As the reactive foods continue to be eaten and absorbed, the body continues consuming body energy, vitamins, and nutrients to maintain the massive immune response necessary to keep the body safe from the consistent ingestion of the sensitive foods.

An example of a common sensitive food in our culture is wheat, more specifically a lectin found in wheat called gluten. Gluten is part of the elastic, rubbery protein found in wheat, barley, oats and rye. It is the part of the grain that binds the dough in baking. Flours that do not contain gluten do not behave in the same way and a binder has to be added in order for it to be used for baking breads, cakes, biscuits, pastry, and pizza. Gluten-rich flour is used widely in the food manufacturing industry as a thickener and cheap filler. Gluten is added to some flours, particularly for bread making, to make them "strong."

Do You Have Food Sensitivity?

Let's take a closer look at hidden food allergies (also called sensitivities) and how they may affect our weight and well-being. Most people think of a food allergy as a dramatic reaction that occurs immediately. But we aren't going to be talking much here about these strong, obvious kinds of allergic reactions to foods. After all, no one gets addicted to foods that close his throat or cause rashes, like strawberries, shellfish, and peanuts. We're talking about food reactions that you are so used to that you may just consider them normal, like bloating, stomachaches, gas, constipation, low energy, joint pain, headaches, earaches, runny noses, postnasal drip, and even ADHD (attention deficit hyperactive disorder). These are some of the most common symptoms of food intolerance or allergy. Ironically, the most "intolerable" foods, the ones most likely to cause these annoying and chronic symptoms are often your very *favorite* foods.

The client's usual response is, how can all of this damage occur without my knowing? The majority of food sensitivity reactions are silent, insidious, and chronic for one simple reason: They take place in the tissues and organs that do not perceive pain or discomfort. Thus, chronic immune assaults can go on daily with no recognized symptoms until our body finally is overwhelmed and develops chronic symptoms. What many clients never realized was that it was possible to be sensitive and have a reaction to any number of foods, but the research shows there are commonly only seven foods that cause this reaction-addiction. They are a small family of grains that includes wheat, rye, oats, and barley; cow's milk; sugar; corn; soy; eggs; peanuts. It is obvious to the food industry that so many people crave wheat products, milk products, and sugar, so it is not surprising to find all three together in many processed foods.

These "sensitive seven" most commonly reactive foods have a unique effect on your brain that can make them impossible to resist. As with alcohol and drugs, the first taste can lead to trouble every time—if you are sensitive to these foods. Not every individual will be affected in the same way by each reactive food, but a particular food seems to result in the same symptoms each time it is eaten by the same individual.

We know now that the body tries to calm the irritation caused by allergy foods by releasing powerful, soothing chemicals. Chocolates and candy loaded with sugar, yogurt and cream cheese made from milk, and grain-based foods like pasta and cereals can set off powerful drug reactions in your brain, if you are sensitive to them. Sugar consumption can trigger a brain release of the powerful painkillers, the endorphins.[1] Casein, the protein in cow's milk, and gluten, a protein found mostly in the grains wheat, rye, oats, and barley, stimulate the production of exorphins, opiate chemicals very similar to endorphins.[2] Over time, these pleasurable brain chemicals can become heavily addicting. If you don't have your doughnut with your coffee and cream, you won't get that feeling of comfort that you like so much.

In fact, when I had clients who had reached plateaus who had given me a food log, it was common for me to see one or more of the "sensitive seven" foods with each meal. At first I would suggest they give up the wheat and dairy for a couple weeks because in my experience these tended to be the biggest metabolic offenders. Many of you reading this probably already know how hard it can be to "withdraw," especially if you are addicted to more than one of these seven reactive foods but for many clients they had never put two and two together. Many of the clients found by avoiding these foods for a short period of time and then reintroducing them back into their diet, the cravings returned, they began overeating these foods again, and started feeling guilty, with mood swings that had disappeared now returning along with the weight they had lost.

Could Reactive Foods be the Cause of Weight Gain?

The likelihood of food sensitivities in individuals who are overweight is strong, if not certain. The very nature of overweight suggests an inappropriate response to food since it is not uncommon to find overweight people who eat less food and exercise more than would be indicated by their body fat. Rather than insinuate that a person is confused about the volume of food he or she eats, medical professionals should conduct food-sensitivity testing to detect any reactive foods. By eliminating these foods, people who test positive for food sensitivities can resume a "normal" weight loss appropriate for calorie intake and exercise.

In fact, for many clients who were conscientious enough to avoid the obviously fat-building foods such as refined sugars found they could often achieve the same peaceful state by eating (or overeating) pasta, bread, cereal, or any number of refined "low-fat" or "no-sugar" foods. The dilemma is processed foods that enhance serotonin also stimulate other body hormones such as insulin. The end result is that the more one eats for the serotonin effect, the fatter one gets.

Sadly the serotonin effect is, in the case of food sensitivities, temporary at best. When you eat a food to which you are sensitive, you stress your body, actually creating a decrease in serotonin in the eating center of the brain, but not necessarily immediately. For example, say a person is sensitive to corn. If she eats a food sweetened with high fructose corn syrup, or even a corn chip, the immediate result may be a familiar reaction in the body resulting in increased serotonin. Concurrently, however; the food may activate the immune system, resulting in various other chemical reactions depending on the immune system response to the food.

A food that is generally healthy for you can, a week later, set up a cascade of immune and chemical reactions in your body that have far-reaching implications if left undiagnosed. The more frequently you eat this food, the greater the strain on your systems and organs until physical symptoms may take you to your doctor. Baffled by your otherwise good health, your doctor will treat your symptoms as indicated. Unless he or she considers food sensitivities as a possible cause and does appropriate testing, your symptoms are destined to return as you continue eating the culprit food. After an appropriate number of visits, your doctor will add the adjectives "chronic" or "recurrent" in front of your original diagnosis. He or she will do further tests, change your medication, and console you in that you may require continued treatment for this problem for which there is no apparent cure.

This is the plight of many of the clients I have seen over the years - they deal with their migraine headaches, sinus drainage, ear infections, overweight, irritable bowel syndrome, chronic fatigue, arthritis, and fibromyalgia, just to mention a few. All these "conditions" may be merely symptoms of a body's defense system mistaking a normal food for a dangerous invader. It is to your body's credit that this protective mechanism exists and works. Unfortunately, your body uses incredible amounts of energy to protect your immune system and subsequently your organ systems when it is switched on inappropriately.

When your immune system is continuously stressed, protecting you from this food that keeps reappearing, it can no longer maintain its defenses against true invader viruses and bacteria. Likewise, nutrients otherwise destined to support other organ systems are recruited by the immune system to support its functions. This sets in motion another cascade of events that may eventually result in symptoms of "malnutrition" or deficiencies in nutrients. As each organ system is taxed by the immune system, it may present symptoms that complicate health.

Unless you're doctor is insightful enough to consider food sensitivities as the root cause of all your symptoms, your array of diagnoses can be numerous. Each may require medical visits and medication to control symptoms. Americans are not given to dealing with problems for the long term and our medical system struggles to live up to our expectations because we are addicted to instant gratification. As depression and frustration take over the individual's daily life, they often become a willing subject of the medical system that seems to be the only hope.

What is the Role of Exercise in Food Sensitivity?

Exercise can become frustrating when you consume little or no healthy fats for energy and become hungrier from your daily exercise. When fat is not accessible to burn for energy, the body falls back on its emergency supply: the small glycogen store in the liver and muscle. Once this readily available source is used up, the body will send a signal for you to eat as quickly as possible.

If the biochemical reaction precipitated by food sensitivity blocks your metabolism of fat for energy, you repeatedly tap your emergency carbohydrate supply. Your body then insists you eat to replace this supply, and odds are slim that you will make a healthy and natural carbohydrate choice. You are more likely to consume easily available processed food loaded with refined sugar and refined (fake) fats.

Eventually, just as I have seen with many clients and friends, this continual cycle of living off your emergency supply of carbohydrate results in a slow but steady buildup of fat storage and the feeling of total dependence on carbohydrates for energy. The next step is usually to stop exercising altogether out of the frustration of seeing all that time and energy not producing any results.

Is False Fat to Blame?

In the book, The False Fat Diet, Elson M. Haas, M.D. shows how food sensitivities strongly contribute to several disorders of metabolism. Below is a step-by-step process that is outlined in the book that details the potential cycle that can be created by the "sensitive seven" foods we mentioned earlier in this chapter. Dr. Haas calls it, The False Fat Phenonenon: the Fat-Creating Cycle of Food Reactions:

1. Eating reactive food
2. Serotonin drop. Blood sugar drop. Adrenaline drop. Endorphin Drop.
3. Mood alterations, including anxiety, compulsive urges and onset of depression.
4. Cravings for and bingeing on reactive foods and high carbohydrate foods.
5. Immune and hormonal reactions, leading to tissue swelling and bloating.
6. Feeling of heaviness and fatigue.
7. Storage of excess food calories, primarily as fat.

8. Decline in metabolism and thermogenic fat-burning capability.
9. Further fatigue, mood deterioration, and weight gain.
10. Continued cravings, and ingestion of more reactive foods.
11. Inflammation and swelling of intestinal membranes, allowing assimilation of allergens and deterring assimilation of healthy nutrients.
12. Nutrient deficiencies which weaken immune function and heighten disease processes.
13. Candida yeast colonization and infectious disorders.
14. Inflammatory changes in the intestinal lining, from yeast irritation, increased swelling and bloating, more fermentation of foods and increased digestive impairment.
15. Increased reactivity to foods and increased cravings.

From the above cycle we can see how many of our clients face an uphill battle if they continue to consume foods that have the potential to interfere with the hormonal balance of the endocrine system, including the thyroid and adrenal glands. This makes it harder for the body to burn fat. These foods also disturb insulin levels, even in people who are able to maintain normal function of the thyroid and adrenals. This signals the body to convert food energy into fat, and also contributes to hypoglycemia. Including the above mentioned mood chemistry disruptions. When you add all this together, you interfere greatly with the ability to exercise – another reason to choose your food wisely.

How to Test for Trigger Foods?

In the book, *Your Hidden Food Allergies Are Making You Fat* by Rudy Rivera, M.D., and Roger D. Deutsch you will learn about the revolutionary ALCAT Test, which pinpoints your personal "trigger foods" – foods as common as oranges or wheat – that are causing you to stay overweight. The authors point out that by simply eliminating those trigger foods, you will lose weight and regain your energy naturally.

"After using the ALCAT food sensitivity test extensively, one cannot help but be impressed with its accuracy and versatility. It doesn't simply measure your level of a blood constituent and leave your doctor to figure out what might be causing this abnormality. This form of blood test specifically quantifies the response of your blood to a specific food. The ALCAT Test is itself the diagnosis and prescription for treatment—the best of all worlds," says Dr. Rivera.

In the ALCAT Test, the "normal" used to standardize the results is your own blood and cells. Thus a normal test is what's normal for you, as opposed to your being compared to a group of strangers. In other words, if you test strongly positive to a food, your treatment is to avoid that food. Cut and dried: simple test, simple treatment. In our day of incredibly complicated tests and interpretations, having a blood test that tells all is a relief.

As Dr. Rivera says, "to oversimplify the value of this straightforward test would be difficult. Sometimes this raw truth can intimidate patients, who are accustomed to a medical system that often hedges rather than commit to a diagnosis and treatment. Patients are often shocked to find they are reactive to their favorite foods and the recommended treatment is to simply stop eating them."

After the initial shock wore off for many of Dr. Rivera's patients, they were ready to make a rational plan to begin eliminating foods. Depending on the number of reactive foods involved, many of his patients begin by eliminating a few of the most frequently eaten foods. After a week or two they should add a few more foods to their elimination list until all are included. "However, they must eliminate all reactive foods to confirm whether food intolerance is or is not causing a symptom. Losing weight by spending money on eating the right food is certainly better than spending money on medication," says Dr. Rivera.

Bettina Newman, R.D. points out an interesting weight loss study using the ALCAT Test that was conducted at Baylor Medical College in Texas in her article, Is A Hidden Food Allergy Making Your Fat. The study demonstrates how the removal of the "offender" foods from the diet can result in weight loss. One hundred subjects were divided into two groups. The experimental group followed individual diet plans based upon the results of the ALCAT Tests; members of the control group pursued their own choices of weight-loss plan. After a month, the experimental group dropped significantly more pounds and a greater percentage of body fat. They even increased lean body mass (the ratio of muscle to fat).[3] Investigators in a Spanish study corroborated these results.[3]

What Does The Research Say?

Does the Blood Type Research work? What Dr. D'Adamo has learned from collecting thousands of certified medical results from readers and patients is that it works for nine out of ten people and that the more severe the problem, the faster it works. But the real question each person needs to ask is, "Does it work for me?" It is not as important to have a theory that works for everybody in a generic way as it is to have a theory that takes into account individual variations.

In the years since the publication of the book, *Eat Right 4 Your Type*, Dr. D'Adamo has communicated with hundreds of thousands of people during media appearances, on the Web, over the phone, by mail, at lectures, and in his office. Many of them have been curious, a few skeptical, and some true believers in the Blood Type Research.

On Dr. D'Adamo's Web site **(www.dadamo.com)**, people share, with touching detail, their long efforts to find a key to a chronic illness or a battle with obesity. Their stories have common elements, but at the core they are utterly unique and individual - just like the individuals themselves. This has helped Dr. D'Adamo appreciate more than ever before the countless variations among humans.

You will find no absolutes in the book. The Blood Type Research has never been about rigid rules and regulations. Nor is about superimposing an artificial set of values on the way you already live. Eating right for your blood type simply means following the ancient codes that are still imprinted in every cell of your body.

Even before Dr. D'Adamo's book *Eat Right 4 Your Type* was published there were doctors using the "D'Adamo Serotype Panel 1 (DSP-1) for blood testing with results that included a food list determined by parameters Dr. D'Adamo had programmed into this test. This list was intended for use by the physician in making final dietary suggestions after incorporating as many other factors (such as allergy testing) as they saw fit.

So, knowing of patients who were getting results with weight loss as a side effect of using this system, because most of the patients I had been aware of were using this system for allergies, asthma, arthritis, gastrointestinal inflammation, helped me became aware of the effects that wheat gluten and milk casein were having as contributing factors in the majority of these conditions.

I had learned of the effects that specific foods had on the body systems that control weight depending on your blood type. Certain foods were shown to:

1. Inflame the digestive tract lining
2. Interfere with the digestive process, causing bloating.
3. Slow down the rate of food metabolism, so you don't efficiently burn calories for energy
4. Compromise the production of insulin.
5. Upset the hormonal balance, causing water retention (edema), thyroid disorders, and other problems.

For the client who on the surface looked to be doing everything right but still at a plateau, I would suggest applying the principles in the book, *Eat Right 4 Your Type* as a therapeutic tool and not as a rigid way to live their life. It has always been my approach to leave no stone unturned and through all the clients that I witnessed breaking through plateaus using this research, it became clear they could not all be exceptions to the rule or be discounted as just the result of the placebo effect.

What Can You Do?

A habit is something you don't know you're doing. Once you know you're doing it, it's not a habit anymore - it now becomes a choice and normally it is a conscious choice. So, after gaining this new found awareness of watching these reactions take place in response to the sensitive foods, preventing a repeat would seem straightforward enough—avoid and remove the problem foods. By avoiding these foods, you can potentially remove these reactions and possibly eliminate the cost of treating a chronic medical condition. Rather than buying medication and keeping doctor appointments for the rest of your life, you simply stop eating your reactive food or foods for a period of time.

Often, after four to six weeks, you will see a difference, but some individuals may need up to three to six months, and after that time you can begin reintroducing these foods into your diet if you wish. The key is finding your individual tolerance level for those foods and working with your body. All in all, you save instead of spend money to cure this condition. You stop buying your reactive foods, you add new foods to your diet, and you learn the most basic of lessons: Your health is *your* responsibility. No one knows your body better than you do.

As for milk allergies, if you eliminate milk products from your diet as we have stated above and then after a period of time you then reintroduce them and find your nasal congestion or stomach problems come back along with your cravings, try eating only lactose-free milk products or taking a broad spectrum enzyme supplement that contains lactase. If you still have bad reactions, it's time to move on to milk products derived from goats or sheep instead of cows. If you react to those foods, then forget about trying to consume milk products and look to rice or almond milk as an alternative. However, you may find that cottage cheese, aged cheese, buttermilk, and yogurt are easier to digest because they are already partially digested by being cultured.

As far as wheat goes, there are gluten alternatives. Essene and Ezekiel breads (found in health food stores and in the health food section of your grocery store) are 100% sprouted wheat breads; the gluten lectin is destroyed in the sprouting process. Spelt Bread is a wheat alternative without the gluten. 100% rye bread can be an alternative for blood types O, A, and AB, but the rye lectin can still be an issue for type B. There are many wheat-free / gluten-free pastas (including rice pasta) that are also available. Remember, even wheat-free alternatives can be troublesome, if eaten often enough, when attempting to burn excess body fat because excessive carbohydrates increase blood levels of insulin. Insulin is a fat-storage hormone that converts those carbohydrates into stored body fat.

What's Your Next Step?

Just as no single mechanism lies behind all food intolerance, no two people with food intolerance are the same. For one thing, an aspect of genetics, called genetic polymorphism, affects all types of reactions that might be associated with symptoms caused by food. Genetic polymorphism is what makes each of us different, despite the fact that our genetic makeup is almost identical. This means that distinct types of factors are uniquely common to a group of people within the human race—for example, Europeans, or American Indians. These groups have different enzymes or enzymes that operate at a unique rate. If your ancestors were never exposed to a particular food, it's likely you and others in your group never developed a genetic predisposition to deal with it enzymatically. As such, it has been discovered that different groups will react to food, its metabolism, and its toxicity in different ways.

Numerous scientific studies have demonstrated the effectiveness of identifying and then avoiding foods to which one's body reacts poorly and increasing numbers of physicians, nutritionists and other health care providers believe that the body's physiological reaction to foods, irrespective of their nutritional content, may sometimes be responsible for excess weight. "Food allergy clearly affects the majority of the American people," declares James Bradley, M.D., author of *Dr. Bradly's Food Allergy & Nutrition Revolution.*

What researchers are finding is that each individual's biochemistry is completely unique. Although primarily inherited, it is also affected by environment, lifestyle, health, and other experiences. As such, each person with food intolerance has different symptoms, which vary in degree, age of onset, duration, location, and amount of food needed to trigger the symptoms. The same food can produce vastly different symptoms in different people, and different foods can cause different symptoms in the same person. So, before you have eaten even one mouthful of food, several scenarios are possible. These factors explain why no one single diet will fit every person's nutritional and health needs. Just this awareness alone, of which foods can be reactive for you and minimizing these effects, will help ensure that allergens and toxins that interfere with maximum health do not overload your system.

It's important to remember that when we are sick, many times it is just the body's way of cleansing itself and flushing the impurities from the system. So, as you read through this book, you get a clear understanding of the multitude of problems that can occur in our digestive system, immune system, and enzymatic system. When any one of these systems are not working, a person has taken a step further away from optimal health. The aim of maximum health is to get these processes and others working at optimum performance.

Once you get these systems healthy, you've taken a giant step toward enabling your body to use these dynamic and powerful systems to take care of themselves. Clearly, if you remove food to which you are intolerant, you'll give your body a fighting chance to clear up the migraines, joint pains, excess weight, and other health problems triggered and compounded by foods. Identifying and removing reactive foods is the key to your good health.

CHAPTER TEN

CHANGING YOUR BELIEFS
ABOUT WEIGHT LOSS
BY PATRICK K. PORTER, PH.D.

Changing Belief Systems About Weight Loss

When Martin Luther King, Jr. made his famous speech, I Have a Dream, he used words to create visual images that stirred the emotions of everyone who heard them. Notice what happens in your mind's eye and in your body as you read the following excerpt from that speech:

> *"I have a dream that one day on the red hills of Georgia, the sons of former slaves and the sons of former slave owners will be able to sit down together at the table of brotherhood.*
> *I have a dream that one day even the state of Mississippi, a state sweltering with the heat of injustice, sweltering with the heat of oppression, will be transformed into an oasis of freedom and justice.*
> *I have a dream that my four little children will one day live in a nation where they will not be judged by the color of their skin but by the content of their character.*
> *I have a dream today!"*
> *Try this quote from George Washington on for size.*
> *"If the freedom of speech is taken away then dumb and silent we may be led, like sheep to the slaughter."*

What kind of mental image do you get from the President's statement? How does it make you feel?

Here is one more from John F. Kennedy. Again, notice the images created in your mind and the emotions those images stir:

Chapter 10 | Changing Beliefs About Weight Loss

"Let the word go forth from this time and place, to friend and foe alike, that the torch has been passed to a new generation of Americans - born in this century, tempered by war, disciplined by a hard and bitter peace."

George Washington, John F. Kennedy, Martin Luther King, Jr., and other great leaders like them were able to move our nation and the world to action because of their amazing ability to stir our emotions through visual images. This is the world-changing power of creative visualization.

What is Visualization?

When we see with the mind's eye, we are visualizing. For example, when was the last time your mind drifted away from an activity and into a daydream? If you're honest with yourself, it probably happened within the last hour. In fact, it may have happened while you were reading this book. Daydreaming is normal; everyone does it, though some people are better at it than others, and others are more frequent visitors to their internal world. Daydreams generally happen in pictures, not words. The same is true with visualization. Visualization uses your internal perceptions to create specific visualized scenarios.

Most people habitually create negative images and think negative thoughts rather than positive ones. Dieters are often experts at this. They see themselves as fat, they fantasize about food all the time, and they focus on everything they can't have rather than focusing on what they can have. On top of all that, they envy the thin people in their lives. One overweight client once said to my wife, "You're so thin, I hate you!" How will she ever create a slender body for herself if she hates thin people?

Conversely, naturally thin people see themselves slim and healthy, think of food as nourishment, and don't give food a thought between meals. If you are a chronic dieter, this book will help you break that pattern so you can think and behave like a naturally thin person. Now wouldn't that be easier?

For most people, visualization is the primary component of the imagination. Albert Einstein was by no means the only great mind to use visualization. Many of history's inventors and artists attribute their success to an exceptional ability to visualize. Thomas Edison, Nikola Tesla, Henry Ford and the great composer, Chopin, all claimed to have used creative visualization to spark their imaginations.

I believe that thoughts are the most powerful force in the universe. Everything begins with the mind. All the amazing technology we take for granted today—cars, computers, cell phones, televisions, even everyday items such as cups and eating utensils—started with someone's thought.

To better understand visualization, try thinking about one of your favorite childhood experiences. Notice the images that come into your mind as you mentally relive that event.

Now remember a time when you accomplished something that made you proud of yourself. What images do you see with your mind in this experience? What feelings do you get from the experience? These are examples of visualizing from memory.

Now imagine an upcoming event. Perhaps you have plans to attend a wedding, birthday party, or concert. Choose one occasion and then let your mind conjure up images of what you expect to happen. What images do you see with your mind in this experience? What feelings do you get from the experience? These are examples of visualizing from imagination, and this is the primary type of visualization you will be using during the upcoming "thought experiment."

CHAPTER 10 | CHANGING BELIEFS ABOUT WEIGHT LOSS

Humanity's ability to create and innovate arises from our ability to visualize from imagination. Additionally, this kind of imagined visualization has long been the primary tool for mind/body healing. From a scientific perspective, we know that, because visualization directly impacts the body's neurological system, it can have a direct influence on us physically.

Imagine I have just handed you a large, yellow, juice-filled lemon. You slice the lemon into quarters and bring one of the quarters to your mouth and bite into it. What happened? Did your mouth begin to pucker? Did it fill with saliva? This is a naturally occurring neurological response to an imagined thought.

Have you ever watched a horror film and, in the midst of the excitement, found your palms sweating and your heart pounding? You knew it was "just a movie," though, right? This is another example of how your body is affected by what's happening in your mind. Here is another scenario that demonstrates the power of mind over body:

You walk down a hallway toward your office. You're feeling sharp in a brand new outfit. Your shoulders are back and your head is high. A co-worker stops you to chat. "You okay?" the co-worker asks. "You look like you don't feel well."

"I'm fine," you say. Your shoulders slump and you return to your office. What did your co-worker mean? Maybe you're just tired. Or maybe you really are sick. Maybe you need that facelift after all!

After lunch the same co-worker meets you in the hall. "Are you sure you're okay?" she asks. "You look pale today." By mid-afternoon, you're exhausted and your body aches. Work is a chore. You'd give anything for a nap. Maybe you should go home and rest.

Most of us have had a similar experience—where one simple suggestion changes our entire mood and the way we feel physically. Of course, now that you are aware of this mind/body connection, you can change everything. If someone tells you you're not looking well, you can simply gauge the way you feel and know when the person is off base. Something as simple as bad overhead lighting may be the culprit. Just in case you haven't yet got the idea, though, let's try one more scenario:

You're driving down the highway on a sunny Sunday afternoon. You're singing along with your favorite song on the radio. You're doing the speed limit. Suddenly you hear a siren, and flashing blue lights fill the car. What happens? Does your heart start pounding? Do your palms get sweaty? Does your breathing get shallow?

Why does all this happen even if you know you're doing everything right? Because your mind is conditioned by past experience—or by a kind of social hypnosis—to respond to this particular stimulus with fear, your brain kicks the fight-or-flight response into high gear, and your body responds.
What I want you to understand about the mind/body connection is this: If the mind can have this kind of impact on the body, is there any reason the mind can't also be harnessed to overpower the effects of nicotine, stimulate the metabolism, trigger the immune system to eliminate unwanted cancer cells, or do away with pain?

Why Creative Visualization?

Creative visualization, otherwise known as guided imagery, uses language to transport individuals out of their current space and into a new space of inner calm, peace, and tranquility. A natural byproduct of creative visualization occurs when the muscles go loose and limp, thereby creating the relaxation response. When we use creative visualization to changes unwanted habits, we call it *behavioral repatterning*.

What is the Relaxation Response?

In the late 1960s, in the same room in which Harvard Medical School's Walter Cannon performed fight-or-flight experiments fifty years earlier, Herbert Benson, MD identified a counterbalancing mechanism to the stress response. In his research, he discovered that, just as stimulating an area of the hypothalamus could cause a stress response, activating other areas of the brain results in stress reduction. He termed this opposite state the relaxation response.

Once the relaxation response is triggered, the brain sends out neurochemicals that virtually neutralize the effects of the fight-or-flight response. We immediately notice the physical benefits such as a decrease in blood pressure, a lower respiratory rate, a slower pulse, relaxed muscles, and an increase in alpha brainwave activity. I'll discuss the importance of brainwaves in an upcoming chapter. For now, just know that alpha brainwaves are associated with deep relaxation and being in this state allows for greater access to what I call the intuitive mind, which is where overcoming unwanted eathing habits is most likely to take place.

Because the relaxation response is hard-wired, you do not have to believe it will work for you to experience the benefits. The relaxation response happens in the body and not in the mind. As you read, you will learn in detail how to turn on the relaxation response, which naturally turns off the harmful fight-or-flight response, so you can easily transform your life and your world. The relaxation response is the perfect state for learning, healing, or focusing on your weight loss goals.

"Repeated activation of the relaxation response can reverse sustained problems in the body and mend the internal wear and tear brought on by stress."

-Herbert Benson, MD
Timeless Healing, 1996

Why use Creative Visualization and Guided Relaxation Together?

We all have an inner critic, a part of our mind that, based on past experience, will reject new information without proper evaluation. This is known as the critical factor. Relaxation techniques subdue the critical factor of the mind. In other words, the part of the mind that might reject unfamiliar information is put on hold during the relaxation response.

Everyone possesses a right-brain and a left-brain. These two parts of the brain play a role in your eating habits and are essential components in creating lasting lifestyle changes.

What's the right-brain got to do with it?

The right-brain is the creative part of our nature and is capable of visualizing incredible things for us. As a child, if you had a more active right-brain, there is a good chance your parents often had to tell you, "Stop daydreaming," or, "Come back to earth." Although the right-brain can help you fantasize what you want, it can also cause you to imagine what you don't want, which won't get you anywhere or will create excess stress in your life. Your mind needs direction.

Even though the brain receives messages from all five senses—sight, sound, smell, taste, and touch—it stores the messages as pictures or symbols. This is why people who rarely engage the right-brain often struggle with visualization or meditation techniques. It's also why I'll teach you to use images and symbols to maximize your mind's potential for giving you what you want.

We use guided visualization and relaxation techniques to create positive and appropriate ways for you to imagine your self-image, your health, or your personal goals. This helps you stay optimistic and motivated toward the changes that bring about success. Throughout the book, whenever I mention behavioral repatterning, I am referring to this powerful combination of creative visualization and relaxation.

What's the Left-brain Got to Do With It?

Let's talk about the left-brain. The left-brain is that part of our brain obsessed with control. It likes sequence and order. It is also the part of the brain that recognizes stress and responds to it. Relaxation can only happen when you release control and allow the left-brain to rest for a while. Even though it may seem counterintuitive to let go in order to gain control, this is exactly what happens during the relaxation response.

When you use behavioral repatterning, you subdue the left-brain while stimulating the right-brain. The idea is to give you a balance, so you can reap the rewards of whole-brain thinking. The visualizations are designed to help you let go of fear, stress, and anxiety and, most importantly, to give you the power of possibility thinking.

Possibility thinking involves using the creativity of your other-than-conscious mind to see even the most improbable solutions that can create long-term positive effects on your life. Possibility thinking puts you in a place of choice. Most people rule out new choices based on past evidence, which is self-defeating. Possibility thinking overcomes this preconditioning and allows you to seek the best possible outcome.

On the opposite end of the spectrum is the person who has limited thinking and can only see the reasons why something should fail, even when there is evidence that it could succeed. Possibility thinkers can see a way to succeed even when the rest of the world says there is no way. People like Bill Gates, Steve Jobs, and Oprah Winfrey achieved outlandish success because they are possibility thinkers. They refused to settle for anything less than exceptional. For you, developing possibility thinking is at the heart of each thought experiment. Is it possible you could be the next great innovator of our generation?

How Will Behavioral Repatterning Help You Reduce Stress and Lose Weight?

Behavioral repatterning can help you change the way you see yourself and your life. Once you have a new image of yourself—as a healthy, happy, optimistic person—your fears and frustrations fade away, your anxiety vanishes, your overeating habits disappear, and you no longer let small things stress you.

In other words, behavioral repatterning makes sure you are focusing on everything that makes you feel positive and optimistic. When your perception of yourself changes from stressed person to easygoing person, you no longer will have tension and doubt. If this happens, can you imagine how motivated and energetic you would feel?

I have made a more than two-decade study of people who are naturally easygoing and resilient. I knew that the key to permanent success was hidden in their underlying psychology. By talking with these people, I discovered a common thread that included a positive self-image, a relaxed, easygoing demeanor, the capacity for seeing the future as bright and full of opportunity, and the ability to leave the past in the past. I realized that learning how to visualize and relax the way these people do could be life changing for anyone who tried it. behavioral repatterning can boost your confidence and finally let you reflect inner health and happiness. behavioral repatterning can help you get back to the way you felt before stress overwhelmed your life. Every day men and women just like you discover the power of behavioral repatterning, in order to lose weight, stop smoking, overcome pain, reduce stress, or otherwise enhance their lives.

People who have medical conditions worsened by stress find behavioral repatterning an invaluable tool in reducing the stress-related effects of allergies, asthma, chronic pain, and arthritis, among others.

How Can Behavioral Repatterning Help You Unleash Your Inner Artist?

A few years ago I worked with a well-known author for overcoming writer's block. She once said to me, "I could be insanely creative if I knew no one else would ever criticize what I write." Her comment seemed odd for a published author, but it got me thinking about how much our fear of judgment holds us back.

So take a moment to ask: If no consequences to my creation existed, if I only had to please myself, if I only had to do what I wanted (within the constraints of safety, harmony, and balance within the world) what would I create? . . . What if there was no judgment?

Judgment is a function of the logical left-brain, which is why your left-brain needs taming—so you can unleash your inner artist and get to know the part of you that is infinitely creative, and that knows there is only an infinite number of ways to succeed at losing weight from any given moment.

Imagine that deep within you there is a Leonardo da Vinci, of whom Sigmund Freud once said, "Leonardo da Vinci was like a man who awoke too early in the darkness, while the others were all still asleep."

How Can You Use Logic As a Lever?

In many cases people use idiot logic to defend their positions. For example, a smoker, who has seen irrefutable evidence that smoking could kill her, may still say she can't stop smoking because she's smoked for twenty years. This makes no sense. If you took the wrong way to work for twenty years and then one day found a shortcut with less traffic where you could see more beautiful scenery, wouldn't you immediately stop taking the wrong way? Twenty misguided years wouldn't stop you from taking a more logical route.

Here's another form of idiot logic that one of my weight-loss clients once said: "I can't exercise because I've never exercised before, and now I'm sixty-years old, so it's too late."

"If I told you there was a multi-million-dollar vein of gold twenty fee beneath your feet, would you not dig the hole just because you're sixty and have never dug a hole before?" I asked her.

I once knew a massage therapist who leased space in my office. She and I had become friends, and we would frequently sit and chat at the end of the day.

"I have to make a decision," she said to me one day, "and it's driving me crazy. I'm thinking about going back to college to become a physical therapist, but I just can't decide."

"What's the dilemma?" I asked.

"It's going to take me four years," she said. "I'll be fifty by then."

"How old will you be in four years if you don't go back to school?" I asked.

She stared at me for a moment. "What do you mean?"

"Those four years are going to pass anyway. One way or another, you'll get to fifty. The question is, do you want to spend the next four years pursuing your dream, or do you want to arrive at fifty wishing you had?"

She gave no response.

"If you want to do something different, you've got to start making that change today. If you don't go back to school, what will you be doing?"

"The same thing I'm doing now."

"Would that satisfy you?" I asked.

"No." She shook her head, smiled, and stood up.

"Where are you going?" I asked.

"To register." She shrugged on her jacket and started for the door, then stopped and turned around. "Thanks," she said, "I can't believe I couldn't figure that out myself."

Using logic as a lever is what I did in the examples I've given above. The trick is to find out where you might be using idiot logic or where your thinking might be stopping you from making the changes you want in your life. Once you pinpoint the erroneous thinking, you'll know where you need to make the change.

What Can Your Left-Brain Do for You?

Logical and sequential thinking, time, and control are all processed through your left-brain. When you are figuring out a math problem, or are engaged in the process of writing, you are using the left side of your brain. If you are the type of person who is analyzing every word of this book, or loves to solve puzzles or word problems, you are allowing your left-brain to do what it does best. What types of careers do you think people who are left-brain dominant are going to be attracted to?

If you were thinking of your math teachers or professors you are correct. Lawyers who are constantly analyzing the law and arguing it in court are typically left-brain dominant. You would certainly want your accountant to be left-brain dominant. I would hate to think of a tax return filed by an overly creative accountant!

Because of the nature of science, and its logical tests and rigid procedures, scientists are often left-brain dominant. Engineers, who deal with exact blueprints and create things out of nothing, need an active left-brain.

If you were a Vulcan, like Mr. Spock of Star Trek fame, you would have a dynamic left-brain. Like Spock, the left-brain seeks logic; it believes in control and precision. The left-brain is sequential; everything must make sense. Whether you are speaking with another person, working out mathematical equations, balancing your checkbook, or solving a word game, you are using the left-brain.

Also, the critical factor, which is the part of the conscious mind trained to evaluate information based upon past experience, is part of the left-brain's function. Unfortunately, that critical nature of the left-brain tends to reject new ideas before the creative right-brain has the chance to evaluate them.

The left-brain also controls your sense of time. If a meeting is scheduled for 9:00 am, a left-brain dominant person will arrive a few minutes early, whereas a right-brain dominant person may show up at ten after nine (or later), and won't understand why others get frustrated by his or her lack of punctuality. Right-brainers tend to think that time is approximate. Left-brainers are very controlled by time; everything runs on a schedule. For example, they have a specific time for lunch each day—say noon—and they eat at noon, even if they're not hungry. They eat because it's time to eat. Right-brain dominant people eat when they're hungry or when their appetite gets stimulated.

This is why most overeaters tend to be right-brain

dominant. People who are sequentially-oriented, logical thinkers are usually very controlling and are left-brain dominant.

Here are fifteen characteristics of a left-brain thinker. Check the ones that apply to you.

1. ____ Do you like working with facts?
2. ____ Are you more comfortable dealing with data in a precise and exact way?
3. ____ Do you look at problems in a logical and rational way?
4. ____ Do you like working with numbers?
5. ____ Are you interested in the technical aspect of things?
6. ____ Is performance important to you?
7. ____ Do you prefer to analyze facts?
8. ____ Do you prefer traditional ways of thinking?
9. ____ Do you like facts to be organized and orderly?
10. ____ Do you like to work with detail?
11. ____Do you prefer a stable and reliable work environment?
12. ____Do you feel comfortable with procedure?
13. ____Do you prefer security and safety to risk-taking?
14. ____Is the task at hand what's important to you?
15. ____ Do you do whatever it takes to complete it on time?
15. ____Do you prefer people who are practical?

Total: _____ out of 15 apply

What Can Your Right-brain Do for You?

The right-brain is responsible for creativity, dreaming, and imagination. Composing or appreciating music happen in the right-brain. When you draw a picture or paint on a canvas, you are using the creative right side of the brain. Some might even argue that painting your living room is a creative endeavor.

If you have struggled with poetry or creative writing, this might be because you have not allowed your right-brain creative license. Whether you are sculpting, singing, or dancing like John Travolta, you are engaged in a right-brain function. What types of careers do you think people who are right-brain dominant are going to be attracted to?

If your first thought was an artist, you are correct. Other right-brain occupations include poet, dancer, novelist, interior decorator, or musician. Although this by no means is a complete list, it gives you an idea of the type of work a right-brain dominant person would excel in.

Your right-brain is the place of free-spiritedness, dreams, visions, fantasies, fairy tales, freedom, imagination, romance and make-believe. The right-brain has no boundaries or limitations; it is the realm of pure creativity and possibility.

Seventeen Characteristics of a Right-brain Thinker
Check the ones that apply to you.

1. ____ Do you see the whole picture, but not the details?
2. ____ Do you like change and trying new things?
3. ____ Do you enjoy being busy with several things at the same time?
4. ____ Do you have a vivid imagination?
5. ____ Do you rarely accept "the only right answer," but look for alternatives?
6. ____ Do you enjoy a challenge and a risk?
7. ____ Do you get gut-feelings for new ideas?
8. ____ Can you rearrange ideas and put them together into a new whole? (This is known as synthesizing.)
9. ____ Do you like to vary the way you perform your routine tasks?
10. ____ Do you like to find a connection between the present and the future?

11. ____ Do you experience facts in an emotional way?
12. ____ Are you sympathetic and intuitive toward other people?
13. ____ Do you like interaction?
14. ____ Do you make use of figurative language as well as non-verbal communication (body language, facial expressions)
15. ____ Do you feel empathy toward others?
16. ____ Is problem solving often an emotional, not a logical, process?
17. ____ Do you show enthusiasm when you like a new idea?

Total: _____ out of 17 apply

How Are You Wired?

If you are in a place where you can safely stand up, I would like for you to do so. Support your weight on your right leg and rotate the other leg in a circle. Continue moving your leg in a circular motion and spell your name in the air with your dominant hand.

What happened when you started to write your name? Did you find it was easy to spin your leg in a circle, until you started writing your name? Did your leg stop the circular motion and begin to move back and forth? This happens when the left-brain is dominant. The circle is a right-brain function, but writing is a left-brain function. If the left-brain is dominant, it wins.

Were you able to continue spinning the circle, but forgot how to write your name? This happens when the right-brain is dominant because creating a circle is a right-brain function.

If you were able to do both at the same time, congratulations! This is a rare ability. In fact, fewer than one percent of my seminar participants have been able to do both at the same time. This ability is the domain of a fortunate few who naturally function in a whole-brain state.

Whatever you may have experienced during the process, it provides strong evidence that there is an internal power struggle going on within you. This struggle is between the left and right-brain functions. This is why, whenever you perform a new task, the dominant half of your brain automatically takes over, even though it may not be the ideal part of the brain to accomplish the task.

This internal power struggle means that when some of you walked into math or science class you felt uncomfortable. You might have felt out of place. But maybe when you walked into drama or art class you felt comfortable because that's where your brain was most productive. You felt at home. For others, the complete opposite may be true.

Our behaviors become ingrained and anything outside of our expectations often throws us for a loop. For example, have you ever borrowed someone else's car, reached for the gear shift, only to realize it was in a different place? Or switched from driving a manual transmission to an automatic and your left foot kept stepping on a non-existent clutch? Perhaps you reached for the radio and found the knob was in a different place? Over time, you re-learn where everything is and adapt to the situation. But at first it feels awkward.

What I'm going to show you through behavioral repatterning is how to live in harmony with the right and left-brain and become more whole in your thinking.

CHAPTER 10 | CHANGING BELIEFS ABOUT WEIGHT LOSS

Did You Know that You Will Almost Always Get What You Rehearse In Life, Not What You Intend?

As an example, most experts on nutrition encourage you to drink eight to ten glasses of water a day. You're used to drinking eight to ten colas a day. When you reach for the water, it feels as uncomfortable as having the wrong thumb on top. The same thing is true if you are accustomed to having stress in your life. If people conditioned by stress don't have it, they will find a way to create it because that's what feels most familiar.

Imagine the smoker who is conditioned to smoke upon awakening, after a meal, or while driving. Without the proper re-conditioning, the smoker will never become tobacco-free.

Through behavioral repatterning you are going to learn how to change your neurology—to imagine your body and brain working in a different fashion. While practicing behavioral repatterning, your right-brain, the creative part, sends messages to the left-brain that are processed and turned into habits. This is necessary because the left-brain is sequential, ordered, and timely. It's the control center of your habits.

With creative visualization you can let your ingenuity come out to play. Instead of reaching for a soda, you might ask yourself, "What if I enjoyed water as much as I enjoy a soda?" This gives your other-than-conscious mind another option for quenching your thirst. You now have a behavior that is just as immediate and appropriate, but that's a better alternative.

The bottom line is this: What you did in the past doesn't have to be what you do in the future.

What would happen if you were even more creative? What if you trained yourself so that every time you looked at the clock, you reminded yourself to drink a glass of water, take a deep breath, or some other positive behavior?

If you're like most people, you probably look at the clock many times a day. With the proper training, you'd condition yourself to say, "Wow, it's time for a change!" How empowering would that be? You'd really be using both sides of your brain—you'd be in a whole-brain state.

What are the Benefits of Whole-Brain Thinking?

By accessing the whole-brain, you are able to master verbal and nonverbal communication, develop artistic ability, and process information with perfect recall. Quick and easy problem solving is also a key benefit to thinking with your whole brain.

By using both sides of the brain, you are prompting your mind to, as Albert Einstein recommends, "Question everything." You no longer react out of habit, but engage your whole-brain to envision new responses to situations.

Six Major Facts About Whole-Brain Thinking

1. Learning is a mental process.
2. Intended learning occurs when specific information is retrieved from memory in a usable form.
3. Individuals have different learning styles.
4. The more flexible a person is with new information the more useful that information is.
5. Using the whole-brain may require more time in the study phase but is more efficient in the long term.
6. A whole-brain approach must be used to achieve optimum performance outcomes.

Chapter 10 | Changing Beliefs About Weight Loss

What is this Magic Elixir that Can Transform Your Life and the World?

A magic elixir resides right there in your brain. It's the miraculous mixture of chemicals in your brain that cascade through your body whenever you're relaxed, or think a positive thought, or have a happy experience—or whenever you visualize these things. It's the miraculous power within each of us to eliminate the effects of stress, heal our bodies, and enjoy life to its fullest. The magic elixir is created through the power of your other-than-conscious mind and activated by behavioral repatterning to bring you health, vitality, and anything and everything you desire for your life.

People who dare to relax through behavioral repatterning enjoy all of these benefits and more:

- The Relaxation Response replaces the Fight-or-Flight Response.
- The right and left hemispheres of the brain become more balanced.
- Blood flow to the brain increases, resulting in clearer thinking, better concentration, improved memory, and enhanced creativity.
- Serotonin levels increase by up to twenty-one percent, which calms the mind and body and creates an overall sense of well-being.
- Endorphin levels increase by up to twenty-five percent. These are the hormones that flow through the body when we feel happy. Endorphins provide the brain with alertness, are a natural anti-depressant, provide relief from pain, and create pleasurable and loving feelings.
- Twenty minutes of behavioral repatterning can be equivalent to three to four hours of sleep. Consequently, you may find yourself sleeping less, feeling more rested, accomplishing

more, and basically enjoying life more fully.
- Energy levels soar.
- Relationships become more fulfilling.
- Career satisfaction improves.
- A sense of purpose develops.
- The ability to make personal changes, such as losing weight, quitting smoking, ending nail biting or other nervous habits happens faster and easier.
- And last, but certainly not least, one gains a seemingly effortless ability to handle and manage stress.

Most people would pay thousands of dollars for a magic pill that offers these kinds of benefits. With behavioral repatterning, people get these results in just a few relaxing minutes a day. Are you starting to understand why behavioral repatterning is the key ingredient to the magic elixir that can get you everything you want for your life?

The information from this chapter is found in Dr. Porter's book, *"Thrive In Overdrive, How To Navigate Your Overloaded Lifestyle."* Available at www.ZenFramesBRD.com.

> *"The test of a first-rate intelligence is the ability to hold two opposed ideas in the mind at the same time, and still retain the ability to function."*
> **F. Scott Fitzgerald (1896 - 1940),**
> **"The Crack-Up" (1936)**

CHAPTER ELEVEN

Good Fat or Bad Fat, What's The Difference?
Chris Tomshack, DC

Good Fat or Bad Fat, What's The Difference?
By Chris Tomshack, DC

I hate fish. Make no mistake about it. Unless it's yellow perch or walleye, it won't get eaten by me. If it smells like it even came near the water, forget about it. That includes trout, salmon, shark, tilapia, oysters, mussels, clams, and anything else you can think of. The problem here, though, is that I've read the research; and the research points conclusively to one fact. Fish is good for you.

As the CEO of HealthSource Chiropractic, the world's largest chiropractic franchise, which consists of hundreds of clinics across America serving hundreds of thousands of patients that information puts me in a strange predicament. How do I get all those nutrients that fish contains when I can't stand the fish? I can't believe that I'm the only person out there that feels this way about fish. So let me explain why I'm talking about fish and what that has to do with the fats that your body needs.

I've been extremely health-conscious since I was quite young--about the eighth grade. I distinctly remember buying my first weight set. You know the kind, concrete encased in a plastic covering. Right about that time I also started researching vitamins and other supplements. As I got older, my interest merely intensified and I learned more and more about what should and should not go in my body. Little did I know all that research would set the stage for what I do today... and years later, as the owner of four successful practices, I found myself directly responsible for influencing the health of thousands and thousands of patients. Today, that number is in the hundreds of thousands. For me, staying current is of extreme importance and I'm here to pass my knowledge on to you.

What are Essential Fats?

Despite what you may have heard, not all fat is bad fat. There are "good" fats out there that your body needs every day to perform its most basic functions. The good fats are called essential fatty acids. These are fats that your body cannot make on its own. In order to get them, you've got to eat foods that contain them. Before we get to that, let me describe what these essential fatty acids are.

There are basically two different types of fatty acids. The first is omega-3 and the second is omega-6. Right now we're going to focus primarily on omega-3. We're not going to concentrate on omega-6 because most Americans get plenty of omega-6's already. So the omega-3s are the fats that are most important to understand and learn how to incorporate into our lives. These fats are important fats.

Julius Fast wrote in his book **The Omega-3 Breakthrough** (Tucson, Arizona: The Body Press 1987, ISBN 0-89586-625-0) that good fats (essential fatty acids) actually compete with the bad fats. Keeping this in mind, it would make it all the more important to reduce or minimize the amount of bad fats we're ingesting. "Bad" fats include Trans fats and cholesterol, such as animal fat, that we ingest. Therefore, we should consume a higher quantity of good fats to combat the bad fats that we are putting into our system on a daily basis through foods that we're eating. It's also important to note that these good fats actually increase our HDL or what is considered our good cholesterol.

Why Worry About HDL and LDL?

In working with American adults over the years the most common results I see in their blood work is that their HDL (the good cholesterol) is too low and their LDL (the bad cholesterol) is too high. This is inherently unhealthy. The ratio needs to be reversed. Interestingly enough, one of the jobs of

HDL is to actually bind to the LDL and then transport it to the liver where it is broken down and eventually excreted from the body. To put it another way, the HDL actually minimizes some of the damage already done by the bad fats. This concept is so important to understand and put to use in your own dietary regimen because the typical American is getting way too many bad fats and not enough good fats in their daily diet. In all, it's not that hard to change.

There are three main kinds of omega-three fats. The first is ALA (alpha-linolenic acid). The second is EPA (eicosapentaenoic acid). And the third is DHA (docasahexaenoic acid). We'll just refer to them as ALA, EPA and DHA. Just in case you forgot, these fats are the good fats. These omega-3s provide support for the primary systems of our body--including our nervous system, immune system, cardiovascular system and reproductive system.

Why Do Our Bodies Need "Good Fat"?

Millions upon millions of our body's cells are created and die off each second. These good fats, or essential fatty acids, are required for our body to make and repair healthy cell membranes. This is important because a healthy cell membrane is what is required for all our cells to be able to take in new nutrition and get rid of old waste products. These good fats also help our body produce something called prostaglandin. Prostaglandins help our body regulate many things such as blood pressure, the rate at which our heart beats, blood clotting, and even fertility. That makes them pretty darned important. If you don't like fish, a great source of these essential fatty acids, what are you supposed to do? We'll get to that in a moment.

First, let's talk fish. Fish contains a lot of fatty acids. Specifically, fish contain omega-3 fatty acids. Some fish contain more, some less. The more oily the fish, the more essential fatty acids it contains. Anchovies, salmon, albacore tuna, sardines and mackerel are quite oily and therefore contain a great deal of essential fatty acids. The two types of fatty acids that fish contains are DHA and EPA. Fish do not contain ALA. These fatty acids (DHA and EPA) have been directly attributable to lengthening our lifespan and leading a healthier life.

What is ALA and How Can You Get It?

So what about ALA? Since fish doesn't contain ALA, where are you supposed to get this? One easy place would be from flaxseed oil. As a matter of fact, flaxseeds have the highest concentration of linolenic acid of any food; so it's a great place to start. The problem is that most people do not like the taste of flaxseed, me included. For me, they rank right up there with fish on the taste meter. You can relax, though, because amazingly enough you can purchase flaxseed oil at many health food stores and most of the flaxseed oil concoctions have flavoring built-in to mask the flavor. Strawberry and lemon are my two favorites. And typically, about a tablespoonful of the flaxseed oil will meet your daily requirement.

You can find ALA in other foods, such as walnuts, pumpkin seeds, sesame seeds, avocados and soybean oil, among others. A word of warning is necessary here. You'll find the flaxseed oil in the refrigerated compartments of the health food store. It's there for a reason. When you get it home, immediately put it in the refrigerator. If you forget this key step, flaxseed will turn rancid quickly and become very unpleasant. Nuts and seeds also do better if kept out of the heat.

Can Eating the Right Fat Save Your Heart?

The American Heart Association released a statement in 2002 entitled, "Fish Consumption, Fish Oil, Omega-3 Fatty Acids and Cardiovascular Disease," which described the effects of omega-3 fatty acids on the heart and other functions. This stated that omega-3 fatty acids have the ability to:

- Decrease the risk of arrhythmias (which can lead to sudden cardiac death)
- Lower blood pressure
- Decrease triglyceride levels (triglycerides are bad fats)
- Slow down the growth of atherosclerotic plaque (this plaque clogs arteries)

If you don't get enough of these essential fatty acids, or good fats, all sorts of things can backfire in your body. The most commonly cited deficiency of omega-3 fatty acids relates to memory and mental abilities. This alone should make this deficiency quite important to you.

Other problems related to omega-3 deficiency include things such as nerve disturbances-- often referred to as a tingling sensation--strokes, vision or eyesight problems, a decreased immune system, a tendency of the body to form too many blood clots, increased triglycerides and LDL (bad fats), to irregular heartbeat, learning disorders, impaired cell membrane function, itchiness of the front of the lower legs, menopausal discomfort and growth retardation in infants, children and pregnant women.

That's a pretty far-reaching blanket of potential problems resulting from a deficiency in omega-3 fatty acids. Do I have your attention yet?

What Does the Research Say You Should Do?

At this point, you should be seriously considering upping your fatty fish and flaxseed oil intake. In case you haven't arrived at that conclusion yet, let's talk about what some of the research indicates can happen when you have enough omega-3 fatty acids in your body.

1. Coronary heart disease: several studies have found that men and women who eat fish at least once weekly

have a significantly lower death rate from coronary heart disease than people who do not eat fish at least one time per week (1-3). One of the studies followed 1,822 men for 30 years and found that coronary heart disease was 38% lower in the men that consumed at least 1.2 ounces of fish daily than men who did not eat fish. The study also found that myocardial infarction (heart attack) was reduced 67% in the group that ate fish daily. In the Nurse's Health Study, which followed 84,000 women for 16 years, coronary heart disease was between 29 to 34% lower in women who ate fish at least once a week(4). Another study followed 2,445 Finnish women and revealed that those women who consumed a high amount of fish had a 41% lower risk of coronary heart disease than those who hardly ate any fish at all (5).

2. Sudden cardiac death: sudden cardiac death is when a ventricular arrhythmia sets in, causing the heart to stop beating. One large study analyzed 20,000 men for 11 years, and it found that those who ate fish at least once a week had a risk of sudden cardiac death 52% lower than those who ate fish less than once a month(6). Fish lowers sudden cardiac death.

3. Stroke: an ischemic stroke happens when a portion of the brain does not receive enough blood flow for a period of time. In one study, 79,000 women were followed for 14 years. Those women that ate fish at least two times a week had a 52% lower risk of ischemic stroke than those who ate fish less than once a month(7).

4. Alzheimer's disease and dementia: the most common cause of dementia in America is Alzheimer's disease. Alzheimer's disease is essentially plaque forming in the brain. One study showed that men who had a high amount of DHA in their body had a 40% less risk of developing dementia and a 39% decreased risk of developing Alzheimer's disease(8).

5. Rheumatoid arthritis: fish oil supplementation has been

found to significantly decrease the severity and number of painful or tender joints in a person who suffers from rheumatoid arthritis(9).
6. Inflammatory bowel disease: one study found that patients with Crohn's disease (an inflammatory bowel disease) who supplemented with a large dose of fish oil remained in remission over a 12 month period when compared to those who were just given a placebo (10).
7. Depression: large studies across different countries strongly suggest that as seafood consumption rises, the national rates of depression drops (11).

Personally, I have never suffered from any of these maladies. As of this writing, I am 45 years old. I do supplement daily with both fish oil as well as flax seed oil and each year when I have bloodwork done, it looks just like the blood work of a healthy 18-year-old male. What conclusions can you draw from that?

What's the Right Amount For You?

One of the most common questions I've received over the years from both patients as well as doctors is "how do you correctly prescribe dietary changes to ensure the proper amount of essential fatty acids are in a diet"? Personally, I think it is of utmost importance to first determine what type of fish or supplementation you should prescribe before deciding upon how much to eat or supplement with, because the quality of the fish or supplement can influence the quantity and frequency that you should consume.

Many of the fatty fish previously described, which contain good amounts of essential fatty acids, are bottom dwellers. If the fish spends a great deal of time near the bottom of the ocean, it has a higher chance of picking up contaminants such as mercury. Therefore, even if you don't consume the actual fish, these contaminants can be spread into the fish oil itself.

The typical American without any history of coronary heart disease should ingest a variety of fatty fish at least two times a week. They should also include oils that are rich in ALA such as flaxseed oil, soybean oil--along with flaxseed and walnuts. For those patients who already have coronary heart disease, they should consume about 1 g of EPA plus DHA per day, preferably from fatty fish, under the supervision of their doctor. For those patients who need to lower their triglycerides, 2 to 4 g of EPA and DHA per day provided supplementation under their doctors care would be in order.

In America, where we often think "more is better," we must be careful with essential fatty acids. If the patient takes more than 3 g of omega-3 fatty acids through supplementation, they need to make sure that they are under a doctor's supervision, because high intakes of essential fatty acids can cause excessive bleeding in some people.

Adding Essential Fatty Acids to Your Diet.

One thing to remember when consuming essential fatty acids is that high heat, light and oxygen destroy essential fatty acids. For example, nuts that are not roasted or cooked are far healthier than the roasted variety. You can easily find raw varieties of nuts in any health food store. I would also caution you against using flaxseed oil for cooking as it turns rancid when subjected to high heat. Flaxseed oil or extra virgin olive oil can be substituted for margarine or butter in your warm vegetables. This is a great way to get more of such fatty acids.

Sprinkling flaxseed meal on your vegetables or meats can give them a nutty flavor. When you're cooking, another good way to increase your fatty acid intake is to substitute half of any shortening that is called for with virgin olive oil and a little bit of sea salt. It can often yield very favorable and similar results.

A Plan For Those That Don't Like Fish

Remember earlier I explained my distaste for most fish? How am I getting all the essential fatty acids those fishes contain? For those of us who absolutely can't stand the smell, look, taste or texture of fish, we have to rely on supplementation. When taking fish oil supplementation, I think it's a very good idea to absolutely insist that the fish oil that you invest in is micro filtered. The micro filtration helps eliminate heavy metals or other contaminants that might be found in the actual fish itself. Yes, you can buy fish capsules that are cheaper but they are not micro filtered. Spend the extra couple of dollars to get micro filtered fish oil capsules. Your health is worth it.

Incorporating fish oil capsules as a part of your daily dietary regimen makes it so much easier to ensure that you're getting the correct amounts of the essential fatty acids. The same holds true for flaxseed oil. When it comes to flaxseed oil, most of the brands that I have seen simply require one tablespoonful per day. Remember, if you don't like the taste of plain flaxseed oil, you can get the flavored flaxseed oil. It goes down smoothly and your taste buds will thank you.

When it comes to taking fish oil capsules, make sure that your micro-filtered capsules are ingested immediately before you eat a meal. If you are taking three capsules per day, depending on the amount of the essential fatty acids that you need, be sure to take each capsule and then eat your meal. If you take your capsule after you have eaten a sizeable portion of your meal--or worse yet, after you've eaten your meal--you could be in for an unpleasant experience. It's pretty common to be able to taste the fish oil, which many people find distasteful and could keep you from taking the supplements that you need.

Chapter 11 | Fats Your Body Needs and Why – Essential Fatty Acids

Your Next Step

After reading through this information, you've probably come to the conclusion that essential fatty acids, flaxseed oil and fish oil are the magic pills. That just isn't the case. What I have presented to you is a very solid argument on why you should increase the essential fatty acids in your daily diet.

For those of you who like to see proof for yourselves, I would encourage you to log onto the Internet or go to the library and perform your own research. I think you'll be amazed at the results. I was. What's more, once supplementation or an increase in essential fatty acids becomes part of your daily routine, I believe your blood work values will reflect the positive outcomes occurring in your body.

Another thing to keep in mind is that many people who are engaged in a weight loss program often have woefully inadequate levels of essential fatty acids in their diet, making weight loss that much harder. This is especially true for those people who are on a very low calorie diet, such as the types whereby you consume mostly shakes and protein bars for a given period of time to shed the weight faster. If you are currently on a diet, do yourself a favor and get to the store and pick up some high-quality fish oil as well as flax seed oil. Your body will thank you.

When designing the diet regimen for HealthSource Weight Loss Systems, I insisted that essential fatty acid supplementation be a daily part of the regimen. I also insisted that the fish oil capsules be micro-filtered to greatly reduce the chances of any contamination within the oil. You should too.

If you're not on a diet and simply wish to lead a healthier life, the same prescription applies. Do not buy some generic brand of fish oil or flaxseed oil. Insist on high quality. Most importantly, take a necessary step to a better and more healthy body and begin increasing your essential fatty acid intake while decreasing your "bad fat" intake. I believe the changes that can take place in your body may be simply miraculous.

References

1. Kromhout D, Bosschieter EB, de Lezenne Coulander C. The inverse relation between fish consumption and 20-year mortality from coronary heart disease. N Engl J Med. 1985; 312(19):1205-1209.
2. Kromhout D, Feskens EJ, Bowles CH. The protective effect of a small amount of fish on coronary heart disease mortality in an elderly population. Int J Epidemiol. 1995; 24(2):340-345.
3. Dolecek TA, Granditis G. Dietary polyunsaturated fatty acids and mortality in the Multiple Risk Factor Intervention Trial (MRFIT). World Rev Nutr Diet. 1991;66:205-216.
4. Hu FB, Bronner L, Willett WC, et al. Fish and omega-3 fatty acid intake and risk of coronary heart disease in women. JAMA. 2002;287(14):1815-1821.
5. Jarvinen R, Knekt P, Rissanen H, Reunanen A. Intake of fish and long-chain n-3 fatty acids and the risk of coronary heart mortality in men and women. Br J Nutr. 2006;95(4):824-829.
6. Albert CM, Hennekens CH, O'Donnell CJ, et al. Fish consumption and risk of sudden cardiac death. JAMA. 1998;279(1):23-28.
7. Iso H, Rexrode KM, Stampfer MJ, et al. Intake of fish and omega-3 fatty acids and risk of stroke in women. JAMA. 2001;285(3):304-312.
8. Schaefer EJ, Bongard V, Beiser AS, et al. Plasma phosphatidylcholine docosahexaenoic acid content and risk of dementia and Alzheimer disease: the Framingham Heart Study. Arch Neurol. 2006;63(11):1545-1550.
9. Goldberg RJ, Katz J. A meta-analysis of the analgesic effects of omega-3 polyunsaturated fatty acid supplementation for inflammatory joint pain. Pain. 2007;129(1-2):210-223.
10. Belluzzi A, Brignola C, Campieri M, Pera A, Boschi S, Miglioli M. Effect of an enteric-coated fish-oil preparation on relapses in Crohn's disease. N Engl J Med. 1996;334(24):1557-1560.
11. Hibbeln JR. Fish consumption and major depression. Lancet. 1998; 351(9110):1213.

CHAPTER TWELVE

REVERSING THE AGING PROCESS AND WEIGHT LOSS
BY JEREMY BUSCH, DC

Reversing the Aging Process and Weight Loss
by Jeremy Busch, D.C., C.C.S.P., C.S.C.S., C.Ht.

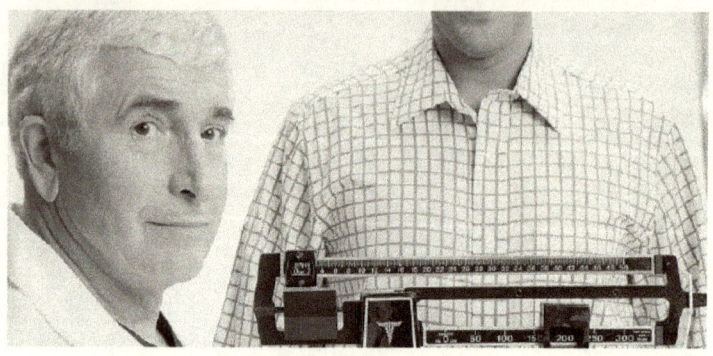

"In this world nothing can be said to be certain, except death and taxes," Benjamin Franklin (1789)

In his letter to Jean-Baptiste Leroy, Benjamin Franklin addressed a very personal subject for modern times.

Death is inevitable. Sooner or later, our tissues will breakdown and cease to operate. Natural death is either a result of chronological age or biological age.

Chronological age is the period that has passed since an individual's exact time of birth. It is like a stopwatch clicking time away at a constant rate of change.

However, biological age is more complex and has more variables influencing the number. The individual's physiology affects how high or low this number is.

This number is influenced by a myriad of environmental as well as genetic variables. According to the "National Vital Statistics Reports" published in April 2009 by the Centers for Disease Control and Prevention (CDC), the life expectancy (chronological age) at birth for 2006 was 77.7 years of age. Further evaluation reveals that 91.23% of the causes of death in United States were a result of a disease or pathological state (Table 1) (Melonie Heron, et al., 2009).

Rank	Cause of Death	Number	Percent of total deaths
	All Causes	2,426,264	100.00
1	Diseases of heart	631,636	26.00
2	Malignant neoplasms	559,888	23.10
3	Cerebrovascular diseases	137,119	5.70
4	Chronic lower respiratory disease	124,583	5.10
5	Accidents (unintentional injury)	121,599	5.00
6	Diabetes mellitus	72,449	3.00
7	Alzheimer's disease	72,432	3.00
8	Influenza and pneumonia	56,326	2.30
9	Nephritis, nephrotic syndrome, and nephrosis	45,344	1.90
10	Septicemia	34,234	1.40
11	Inentional self-harm (suicide)	33,300	1.40
12	Chronic liver disease and cirrhosis	27,555	1.10
13	Essential hypertension and hypertensive renal disease	23,855	1.00
14	Parkinson's disease	19,566	0.80
15	Assault (homicide)	18,573	0.80
	All other causes (residual)	447,805	18.50

Table 1: United States 15 Leading Causes of Death in 2006 (Melonie Heron, et al., 2009)

Almost half of the deaths in 2006 were directly caused by heart disease and cancer alone. In the field of anti-aging medicine, this is a very important trend. If society is in search of a way to delay death and thus increase biological age, elimination or delay of disease is a necessary primary focus. The more healthy someone is, the younger and better they will feel. It's that simple!

"You Are What You Eat"...Yeah!

We have all heard this cliché; however, it is obvious as a nation we have not internalized it. When we take personal accountability of our own diet and health, we can begin to realize the power we have. We can control whether or not we develop pathology. We can control or reduce our own biological age by simply limiting the bad foods and increasing the good foods. According to the CDC, 67% of Americans were either overweight (25<BMI<29.9) or obese (BMI>30) in 2007. The Behavioral Risk Factor Surveillance System from the CDC revealed that only one state had less than 20% of the population as obese. In fact, the state-specific obesity prevalence ranged from 18.7% (Colorado) to 32% (Mississippi). That's obese, not overweight! When you combine the obesity statistics with the leading causes of death, you quickly realize that we are eating ourselves into an early grave!

Western societies have had a complete dietary shift, especially in the last 60 years since the onset of fast-food chains (i.e. McDonald's). We have become such a convenience culture and "need it now" culture that our dietary intake has become mainly processed convenience foods. We have virtually eliminated the intake of fresh fruits, vegetables, lean meat, and fresh fish. In addition, we eat an overabundance of dairy products, cereals/grains, refined cereals, refined sugars, refined vegetable oils, fatty meats, and salt. One study revealed that approximately 72.1% of the total caloric intake comes from these low nutritional, high caloric foods (See Table 2).

As Dr. David R. Seaman states, "The average American consumes about 150 pounds of refined sugar (sucrose and high fructose corn syrup) per year and 60 pounds of refined vegetable oil (margarine, shortenings, and salad/cooking oils) per year." This is enormously out of balance! Not only is this imbalance a leading cause of us becoming FAT, it also has a direct relationship of why diseases like cancer, heart disease, diabetes, Alzheimer's disease, hypertension, arthritis, auto-immune disease, kidney disease, ulcerative colitis, Crohn's disease, Chronic obstructive pulmonary disease (COPD), and other chronic diseases are plaguing Western society. Recent research has demonstrated the overwhelming link between the current Western diet, inflammation, and the diseases previously mentioned (Simopoulos, 1999) (Loren Cordain, 2005) (David R. Seaman, 2002) (Oscar H Franco, 2004).

The pro-inflammatory characteristics of these foods are literally killing us and we need to start taking personal accountability for our own health. Throughout the remaining portion of this chapter these pro-inflammatory aspects of the modern Western society diet are going to be explored. In

Food Group	Value (% of energy[2])
Dairy Products	
Whole milk	1.6
Low-fat milk	2.1
Cheese	3.2
Butter	1.1
Other	2.6
Total	10.6
Cereal Grains	
Whole grains	3.5
Refined grains	20.4
Total	23.9
Refined Sugars	
Sucrose	8
High-fructose corn syrup	7.8
Glucose	2.6
Syrups	0.1
Other	0.1
Total	18.6
Refined Vegetable Oils	
Salad, cooking oils	8.8
Shortening	6.6
Margarine	2.2
Total	17.6
Alcohol	1.4
Total energy	72.1
Added Salt (Sodium Chloride)	9.6

Table 2: Food and Food Types Found in Western Diets (Loren Cordain, 2005)

addition, simple guidelines are going to be outlined to equip every reader with the tools to shift from pro-inflammatory to anti-inflammatory--thus rediscovering the modern "Fountain of Youth".

Inflammation and Prostaglandins:

All inflammation is not bad. In fact, inflammation is a protective mechanism for your body. It has two simple roles: eliminating the cause of the injury as well as repairing any specific damage to the cells as a result of the injury. Without inflammation, cuts would not heal and infections would continue to fester without notice (Ramzi S.Cotran, 1999). Our body needs inflammation to maintain a healthy state.

American society is quite accustomed to dealing with inflammation on a daily basis. Everyone has, at one point or another, taken at least one form of anti-inflammatory medication (i.e. Aspirin, Ibuprofin, corticosteroids, COX2 inhibitors, Vioxx, Celebrex) to reduce or slow the effects of acute inflammation. These medications work by reducing the production of the following very important inflammatory mediators: thromboxane A2 (TXA2), three prostaglandins (I2 (PGI2), F2 (PGF2), and E2 (PGE2)), and two leukotrienes (B4 (LTB4) and C4 (LTC4)) (See Appendix 1) (David R. Seaman, 2002).

The most well known and possibly prevalent is prostaglandin E2. PGE2 has many effects on the body, but all of them are not good. In fact, PGE2 not only increases pain stimulation, but it also increases the degeneration of cartilage and bone as seen in many forms of arthritis and osteoporosis (David R. Seaman, www.deflame.com, 2009). Moreover, it has been directly linked to 12 of the 15 leading causes of death listed in Table 1! When PGE2 either elevates too high or becomes too chronic, it causes the diseases that are killing Americans at an alarming rate. So how do we become "younger"? We learn to control PGE2 through diet.

Fatty Acid Imbalance: Omega 6 vs. Omega 3

In a previous chapter, essential fatty acids (EFAs) were discussed. In this section, two specific dietary EFAs are going to be discussed in more detail: Omega 6 EFAs (i.e. Linoleic acid) and Omega 3 EFAs (i.e. Alpha-linolenic acid). Both are needed in order to sustain health and life. In fact, they have both been a component of the human diet since the creation of mankind. Current research demonstrates that the ratio (balance) of Omega 6 EFAs and Omega 3 EFAs to sustain health needs to be less than a 4:1 ratio respectively in order to eliminate disease.

The problem is that current Western society ingests a ratio of about 20:1 (Simopoulos, 1999)! When more Omega 6 EFAs are ingested, a mass production of disease causing, inflammatory mediators are produced, specifically PGE2. Initially, the levels of PGE2 don't cause any symptoms; however, diseases and symptoms develop after an extended period of exposure to continuing elevated levels of PGE2. A modern society that eats an appropriate ratio of EFA's is the Eskimo society. As a result of eating high Omega 3 EFAs and low Omega 6 EFAs, the prevalence of chronic degenerative diseases, heart disease, diabetes, cancer, appendicitis, diverticulitis, ulcerative colitis, gallstones, psoriasis, multiple sclerosis, and rheumatoid arthritis is virtually zero (David R. Seaman, 2002)!

O6AA: Omega 6 Addiction Anonymous!

Although this is an emphatic statement, many American do actually suffer from a self diagnosed "Omega 6 Addiction." Every meal is over-loaded with Omega 6 EFAs rich foods. Dairy products, cereals/grains, refined cereals, refined sugars, refined vegetable oils, fatty meats, and salt combined are a major component of every meal. At restaurants, bread baskets are given prior to the meal. Sandwiches with inflamed meat (see the next paragraph) stuffed between either white or wheat bread is the staple lunch.

Fried foods (i.e. fish, French fries, potato chips) are consumed virtually daily. Meals are cooked in corn, safflower, sunflower, cottonseed, peanut, or soybean oil. Condiments (i.e. mayonnaise, tartar sauce, margarine, salad dressings, or ketchup) are used in excess to "spice up" the meal. Sugar-rich drinks are consumed in abundance to about 56 gallons per year instead of water (David R. Seaman, www.deflame.com, 2009). In fact, the major color of an American meal is brown! This is Omega 6 heaven! Foods that are rich in Omega 6 EFAs are predominantly grains, pasta, seeds, and sugars. Not only are these foods pro-inflammatory, but they also increase acidity, disrupt blood sugar regulation, and decrease the absorption of calcium, magnesium, and zinc (David R. Seaman, www.deflame.com, 2009).

The US Department of Agriculture (USDA) grades the meat by the "marbling" of fat within the meat. Three categories are Prime, Choice, and Select with the degree of "marbling" decreasing respectively. The inflammatory problem is that the cattle are obese and inflamed from their Omega 6 rich diet (i.e. grain fed). If the cattle are already inflamed from their diet and the meat is consumed, the end result is an inflamed (high PGE2) meal. This isn't exactly anti-inflammatory. What should be sought is either lean meat or wild game. In comparison, grain-fed animals have 20-25% fat by weight versus the 2-4%

fat by weight of wild game. If the cattle are grass-fed instead of grain-fed, the muscle is very lean with most of the fat being stored underneath of the skin instead of within the muscle.

Another benefit is that the meat is high in Omega 3 EFAs due to the cattle diet of vegetables (i.e. grass); therefore, it is anti-inflammatory! It is obvious that grass-fed meat or wild game should be sought as a goal of being anti-inflammatory. A great website to learn more about grass-fed animal products is www.eatwild.com (David R. Seaman, www.deflame.com, 2009)

Set Free with Omega 3:

Welcome to the anti-inflammatory era! Since we have dissected Omega 6 EFAs in detail, we may now proceed to our "Fountain of Youth." The focus of this section is to discuss easy steps on how to switch your diet to an anti-inflammatory diet; thus decreasing the risk of chronic disease. The best way to be successful with this lifestyle change is to make it as simple as possible. The more simple this process, the more success you will experience. In a nutshell, eliminate as many Omega 6 EFAs as possible while increasing Omega 3 EFAs as much as possible by adhering to the following 8 items:

1. **Get Color in Your Diet:** Increase fruits, green vegetables, and nuts. Not only are you increasing Omega 3 EFAs, but you're also going to automatically increase the amount of healthy vitamins, minerals, nutrients, antioxidants, bioflavenoids, and phytochemicals that your body needs to stay healthy and fight disease.

2. **Eat Only Wild Game and Grass-fed animal products:** Two words…ANTI INFLAMMATORY! Grass-fed animal products are rich in Omega 3 EFAs and low in Omega 6 EFAs. What's great is the diversity of products currently available. In today's supermarkets, consumers can purchase grass-fed, lean red meats, fish,

shellfish, fowl, pork, and even eggs rich in Omega 3 EFAs.

3. **Eliminate Grains/Cereals/Pastas:** These increase inflammation, increase acidic body pH, lack nutrients, and promote disease (read the previous section). There is very little benefit from eating grains, cereals, or pastas, but most consumers worry about fiber if they eliminate this category. Current research shows by eating fresh fruits and vegetables, we are getting twice the amount of fiber as whole grains. In fact, broccoli and lettuce are like a turbo-boost of fiber with 8 times the amount of fiber found in whole grains!

4. **Use Extra Virgin Olive Oil or Coconut oil only:** Whenever oil is necessary in cooking, Extra Virgin Olive Oil is a great source of Omega 3 EFAs. If Olive Oil is not available or a "twist" is desired, try coconut oil. These also can be spiced up with vinegar, mustard, or a variety of spices to make a homemade salad dressing or veggie dip! Commercial salad dressings are usually high in sugar and soybean oil; both of which are not anti-inflammatory. Minimal amounts of butter may be tolerated if it is from grass-fed cows.

5. **Drink Water, Water, and More Water:** Water is the only beverage that has absolutely zero negative side effects on the human body. It is also the only beverage that is directly required for optimal health. When thirsty, water should be the main beverage consumed. If variety is needed, green tea may be tolerated in moderation. If an alcoholic beverage is desired, research is showing that red wine and stout beer have anti-inflammatory properties. However, only one serving is recommended to maintain the anti-inflammatory protocols and optimal health.

6. **Use Fruit to Satisfy the Sweet Tooth:** By reaching for a sweet piece of watermelon or strawberries, you

can satisfy most sweet cravings. This is a great way to maintain the anti-inflammatory approach! In fact, many cultures naturally consume fruit at the end of a meal for a "sweet end". Sugary sweets (i.e. pie, ice cream, etc.) are a modern alternative that promotes inflammation and disease. If an alternative is needed, make a "trail mix" of dark chocolate, raisins, and nuts (i.e. almonds) for a nice anti-inflammatory treat. However, eat it sparingly since the dark chocolate and nuts are high in calories.

7. **Exercise:** Exercise is an indisputable method to increase health, increase fat loss, and decrease the risks of chronic diseases. However, this does not mean to immediately go and buy a gym membership. Honestly, keep it simple. Just start walking. The idea is to initially minimize the amount of change as much as possible. If you have a completely sedentary lifestyle, start walking a small amount every other day. If you currently are exercising, great job! Continue what you are doing. Minimizing the amount of change increases your odds of a successful lifestyle change. If you need suggestions of easy activities that burn some calories, see appendix 2. (David R. Seaman, 2002) (David R. Seaman, www.deflame.com, 2009) (Marz, 1999) (R.Seaman, 2007)

8. **Supplement to Optimize Health:** Even with a perfect diet, it is very difficult to maintain the appropriate nutrient levels to maintain health. In fact, current research is now demonstrating the need for supplementation to prevent disease. It can be a very complicated process since there are tens of thousands of potential products. However, we are going to keep to our theme of simplicity. Dr. David Seaman limits his supplementation recommendations to the "core four": a multivitamin, magnesium, EPA/DHA, and coenzyme Q10 (CoQ10). These tend to be the most common supplements that are deficient in the Western diet. Moreover, by consuming these four supplements, energy, antioxidant defense, and tissue healing are all

enhanced while inflammation is directly reduced. How great! The following are the recommended dosage for the core four:

Multivitamin: Dosage depends on the product. However, these are generally a great way to ensure appropriate levels of B-vitamins, minerals, and antioxidants that the body uses for all of its biomechanical processes. It makes the machine function better!

Magnesium: The optimal dosage is from 400 – 1000 mg per day. Magnesium is also directly used in over 300 metabolic reactions within the body. The main problem with Magnesium is diarrhea at high levels of ingestion. There are a few drug interactions, so it is recommended to consult with your physician prior to supplementing.

EPA/DHA (aka Fish Oil): These are the fabulous Omega 3 EFAs! They are great! The recommended dosage is 1-3 grams per day. By supplementing, we can gain more control over the Omega 6 EFAs and Omega 3 EFAs ratio. We can come closer to the recommended 4:1 ratio that is recommended for anti-inflammatory conditions. The only risk is for individuals taking strong blood thinners (i.e. Coumadin) since it can provide additional "thinning" which may cause a problem. Again, consult with your physician prior to use.

Coenzyme Q10: This is becoming more and more popular as more research is being performed on its many benefits. It is currently being used therapeutically for conditions such as congestive heart failure, muscular dystrophy, chronic fatigue syndrome, breast cancer, headaches, and Parkinson's disease to name a few. A major problem is that the production of CoQ10 within the body decreases with age. Therefore, we need to supplement 100 mg per day or more (David R. Seaman, www.deflame.com, 2009) (Marz, 1999) (R.Seaman, 2007).

115 Pound Weight Loss in 7 months:

To see how simple it can be, here is an empowering testimonial from a 36 year old male named Tom. In 2001, Tom was diagnosed with a neurological condition called Cervical Dystonia or Spasmodic Torticollis (ST). This condition can be severely painful with intermittent or sustained muscle spasms in the neck or back. At the time of diagnosis, he was about 185 pounds with an athletic build. Over the next 6 years, he battled depression, panic attacks, and disability to the point of becoming almost completely homebound. Obviously, his weight began to increase. In December of 2006, He was tipping the scales at about 310 pounds (BMI 39.8). That was an increase of 67.6% of his original body weight within 5 years! Now he was starting to notice the toll he was placing on his body. In fact, he was placed on prescription blood pressure medicine for hypertension when he crossed the 240 pound mark. In December 2006, he decided to take control again. Due to his ST diagnosis, it was extremely difficult for him to exercise, but this did not deter him.

Tom became very focused on his anti-inflammatory nutritional guidelines www.deflame.com by limiting pro-inflammatory foods. His diet consisted of an abundance of fresh fruits and vegetables with a modest amount of protein. Usually for dinner, he would either have chicken, fish, steak, pork tenderloin, or lean beef. He eliminated pro-inflammatory foods like bread, pasta, grains, or sweets, and he began drinking only water. If he needed a snack, he would eat a piece of fruit. It was that simple! The only exercise he was performing was walking. He started at ¼ mile a day and gradually progressed to 3 miles twice a day within 3 months. Tom states, "I just make sure that when I eat, I eat the right kinds of food.

When I feel full, I simply stop eating." SIMPLE! There were no confusing diets or advanced exercise programs or any miracle pills. Tom simply ate properly and performed what exercise he could. Within 7 months, Tom went from 310 pounds (BMI 39.8) to 190-195 pounds (BMI 23.1)! He lost 115 pounds in 7 months by eating properly and exercising modestly! In addition to his weight loss, he is no longer on hypertension medications, no more panic attacks, and the painful symptoms from ST are decreased significantly! In fact, he is socially active again and no longer virtually homebound! Great job, Tom! (You can read more of Tom's experience at www.deflame.com.

Anti-inflammatory Recipes:

Making the shift from a pro-inflammatory diet to an anti-inflammatory diet does not mean your taste buds will never be stimulated again. In fact, you will begin to notice a whole new world of diversity available to you. To help you start this journey, Dr. Loren Cordain, the leading authority on the Paleolithic diet, has compiled a list recipes that will definitely get your taste buds dancing during any meal! More are available on his website www.thepaleodiet.com/nutritional_tools/recipes.shtml, but here a few of my favorites (Cordain):

Seafood:
Trout Simmered in White Wine Sauce:

2   Trout
2   *tablespoons of olive or canola oil*
1/3 cup minced shallots or onions
2/3 cup minced carrots
2/3 cup chopped fresh mushrooms
1   *cup white wine*
1   *tablespoon fresh thyme*
3   *tablespoons fresh parsley*

Sauté the shallots, carrots, and mushrooms in oil until the shallots are soft. Add wine and seasonings. Simmer for several minutes. Add trout and cook about 6 minutes per side
(*From: Artemis Simopoulos, The Omega Plan*)

Domestic Low Fat Meat Entrees (Beef, Pork, Chicken):
London Broil with Herbs:

London broil beef (1-1 ½ lbs.) trimmed of all visible fat and cut into four pieces
1 tablespoon canola oil
2 minced garlic cloves
2 teaspoons minced fresh rosemary or 1 teaspoon dried
2 teaspoons minced fresh basil or 1 teaspoon dried
2 teaspoons minced fresh thyme or 1 teaspoon dried
Fresh ground pepper

Place meat in shallow dish. Rub both sides with oil, garlic and herbs. Add pepper and let stand for one hour. Prepare barbeque (high heat) or preheat broiler. Cook meat two inches from heat source to desired state (four minutes per side for rare).

Broiled Pork Tenderloin Zesty Rub:

1 minced garlic clove
1 tablespoon paprika
1 tablespoon dry mustard
1 tablespoon ground coriander
1 tablespoon canola oil
1 tablespoon olive oil
1 tablespoon red wine
1 pound of very lean pork tenderloin, trimmed of all visible fat

Mix dry spices and garlic in a mortar and pestle-add in the oils and wine to make into a paste. Rub the paste onto the pork one hour before broiling. Broil port 2 to 3 inches from heat source for about six minutes per side or until it is cooked to desired condition.

Chicken Breasts with Red Pepper Sauce:

2 medium tomatoes, peeled, seeded, and chopped
1 small onion, chopped
1 medium red bell pepper, chopped
1 tablespoon fresh parsley, chopped
1 tablespoon fresh basil, chopped
¼ teaspoon dried thyme
1/8 teaspoon cayenne pepper
¼ teaspoon fresh ground pepper
4 skinless, boneless breast halves, pounded to ¼ inch thickness
2 tablespoons canola oil
½ cup white wine

Combine vegetables and spices in a medium saucepan. Bring to a boil, reduce heat, and simmer 20 minutes. Transfer to a food processor or blender, and puree until smooth. Pour into a small saucepan and keep warm over very low heat. In a large fry pan, heat oil. Add chicken breasts; cook three minutes a side until chicken turns white. Add wince; reduce heat and simmer for 10 minutes. Spoon red pepper sauce on plate and arrange chicken on top.

Barbequed Spicy Honey Chicken:

3 tablespoons honey
2 tablespoons fresh lemon juice
1 tablespoon fresh orange juice
2 scallions, finely chopped
1 teaspoon finely chopped fresh tarragon
1 teaspoon finely chopped fresh thyme
1 teaspoon finely chopped fresh sage
1 teaspoon fennel seeds, toasted and crushed
Freshly ground black pepper to taste
4 boneless, skinless, chicken breast halves (about 1 pound)

In a large bowl combine honey, lemon and orange juices, herbs, scallions, pepper, and fennel seeds. Put the chicken in the bowl and marinate for 1-2 hours. Fire up the barbeque and grill the chicken, turning constantly while basting with the marinade until the breasts are cooked.

Game Meat Entrees:
Roast Pheasant with Fruit and Nut Stuffing:

1 pheasant (2-3 pounds)
Fresh ground pepper
Garlic powder
Olive oil
1 ½ cups freshly squeezed orange juice
½ cup raisins
3 cloves
½ cup dried and coarsely chopped apricots (non-sulfured)
½ teaspoon grated orange peel
1 cup chopped pecans

Preheat oven to 350 F. Wash and dry the pheasant and brush with olive oil inside and out. Sprinkle inside and out with pepper and garlic powder. In a saucepan combine the orange juice, raisins and cloves. Bring to a boil, reduce the heat and simmer five minutes. Strain the mixture, discarding the cloves and reserving the orange juice and raisins. In a mixing bowl combine the raisins, apricots, ginger, orange peel and the nuts. Mix well and use the mixture to stuff the pheasant. Place the pheasant breast up on a rack in a roasting pan, and roast until tender, about 30 minutes per pound, brushing frequently with the remaining orange juice. Place the pheasant on a serving platter and trickle the liquid from the roasting pan over the pheasant.

Vegetable Dishes:
Chopped Jamaican Zucchini

1 medium zucchini squash, chopped

¼ red onion, chopped

½ red pepper, chopped

½ to 1 jalapeno pepper, chopped (to taste)

¼ cup chopped cilantro (or more to taste)

1 small clove garlic, minced

Pinch of ground coriander seed

Dash lemon juice

Toss all ingredients together; adjust seasonings as desired

Salads:
Colorado Spinach Salad:

1 small bunch fresh spinach

12 dandelion leaves

½ cup pink sorrel leaves, loosely packed

1 apple, cored and cut into bite sized pieces

½ cup walnut halves

You may substitute appropriate fresh greens for the dandelion and sorrel leaves. Wash and de-stem spinach. Coarsely chop dandelion leaves, and tear spinach, then toss dandelion, sorrel and spinach together in a stainless steel bowl. Put aside in refrigerator to drain and cool. When drained, pour off excess water and add apple and pecans. Toss with dressing and serve.

<u>*Colorado Spinach Salad Dressing*</u>:

1 tablespoon honey

1/3 cup lemon juice

Fresh ground pepper to taste

1 teaspoon minced fresh tarragon

1/3 cup olive oil

1/3 cup flaxseed oil

Dissolve honey in lemon juice; add pepper and tarragon and stir. Pour this mixture into a cruet, add the oils and shake vigorously to blend.

Fruit Dishes and Desserts:
<u>*Baked Walnut-Cinnamon Apples:*</u>

4 apples

1 cup raisins

¼ teaspoon cinnamon

½ teaspoon vanilla

½ cup water

¼ cup walnuts

Heat oven to 375 F. Core and piece apples with a fork in several places around the center to prevent them from bursting. Mix raisins, nuts, cinnamon and vanilla in a small bowl. Fill center of each apple with this mixture. Place in a glass-baking dish and pour water into pan. Cover with foil and bake about 30 minutes or until tender.

Conclusion:

Western societies are in desperate need of a dietary shift. However, this one needs to be in the direction of anti-inflammation. If inflammation is allowed to continue to run rampant the average life expectancy of the average American is going to decline as time continues to pass. Chiropractic medicine, pharmaceutical intervention, physical therapy, and surgery can all help with the symptoms of pain or dysfunction; however, none of them address the clinical, chronic diet-induced inflammation. Chronic, diet-induced inflammation has been shown to directly influence 91.23% of the causes of death in the United States in 2006. Correcting this underlying diet-induced inflammation does not have to be difficult. In fact, the shift should be easy. By completing 8 simple steps, one can learn to correct any imbalance by simply focusing on a few dietary principles. In return, they will increase their probability of living a healthier, longer life. The stairway to the current "Fountain of Youth" has 8 steps to conquer. The only challenge is when to start.

Works Cited

1. Cordain, D. L. (n.d.). *The Paleo Diet*. Retrieved October 2009, from www.thepaleodiet.com/nutritional_tools/recipes.shtml

2. David R. Seaman, D. (2002). The Diet-Induced ProInflammatory

State: A Cause of Chronic Pain and Other Degenerative Diseases. *Journal of Manipulative and Physiological Therapeutics*, 25, 168-179.

3. David R. Seaman, D. (2009, October). *www.deflame.com*. Retrieved October 2009, from Deflame.com: www.deflame.com

4. Loren Cordain, S. B.-M. (2005). Origins and Evolution of the Western Diet: Health Implications for the 21st Century. *American Journal of Clinical Nutrition*, 81, 341-353.

5. Marz, R. B. (1999). *Medical Nutrition From Marz*. Portland, Oregon: Omni-Press.

6. Melonie Heron, P., Donna L. Hoyert, P., Sherry L. Murphy, B., Jiaquan Xu, M., Kenneth D. Kochanek, M., and Betzaida Tejada-Vera, B., et al. (2009). *Deaths: Final Data for 2006*. U.S. DEPARTMENT OF HEALTH AND HUMAN SERVICES.

7. Oscar H Franco, L. B. (2004). The Polymeal: A More Natural, Safer, and Probably Tastier (Than the Polypill) Strategy to Reduce Cardiovascular Disease by More Than 75%. *British Medical Journal*, 329, 1447-1450.

8. R.Seaman, D. (2007). Nutritional Considerations in the Treatment of Soft Tissue Injuries. In W. I. Hammer, *Functional Soft-Tissue Examination and Treatment by Manual Methods* (pp. 717-731). Sudbury: Jones and Bartlett Publishers.

9. Ramzi S.Cotran, M. V. (1999). *Robbins Pathologic Basis of Disease* (6th ed.). Philadelphia: W.B. Saunders Company.

10. Simopoulos, A. P. (1999). Essential Fatty Acids in Health and Chronic Disease. *American Journal of Clinical Nutrition*, 70, 560S-569S.

Appendix 1

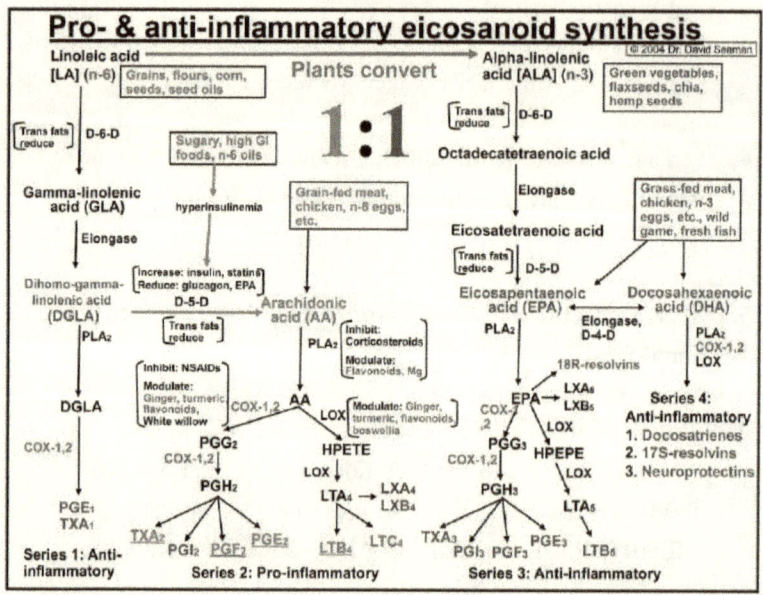

Appendix 2

Activity	kcal/min	Activity	kcal/min
Handball and squash	10.0	Golf: foursome-twosome	3.7-5.0
Mountain climbing	10.0	Horseshoes	3.8
Skipping rope	10.0-15.0	Baseball (except pitcher)	4.7
Judo and karate	13.0	Ping pong-table tennis	4.9-7.0
Football (while active)	13.3	Calisthenics	5.0
Wrestling	14.4	Rowing: pleasure-vigorous	5.0-15.0
Skiing:		Cycling: 5-15 mph (10 speed)	5.0-12.0

Moderate to steep	8.0-12.0	Skating: recreation-vigorous	5.0-15.0
Downhill racing	16.5	Archery	5.2
Cross-country: 3-8 mph	9.0-17.0	Badminton: recreational-competitive	5.2-10.0
Swimming:		Basketball: half-full court (more for fast break)	6.0-9.0
Pleasure	6.0	Bowling (while active)	7.0
Crawl: 25-50 yd/min	6.0-12.5	Tennis: recreational-competitive	7.0-11.0
Butterfly: 50 yd/min	14.0	Water skiing	8.0
Backstroke: 25-50 yd/min	6.0-12.5	Soccer	9.0
Breaststroke: 25-50 yd/min	6.0-12.5	Snowshoeing (2.5 mph)	9.0
Sidestroke: 40 yd/min	11.0	Sleeping	1.2
Dancing:		Resting in bed	1.3
Modern: moderate-vigorous	4.2-5.7	Sitting, normally	1.3
Ballroom: waltz-rhumba	5.7-7.0	Sitting, reading	1.3
Square	7.7	Lying, quietly	1.3
Walking:		Sitting, eating	1.5
Road-Field (3.5 mph)	5.6-7.0	Sitting, playing cards	1.5
Snow: hard-soft (3.5-2.5 mph)	10.0-20.0	Standing, normally	1.5
Uphill: 5-10-15% (3.5 mph)	8.0-11.0-15.0	Classwork, lecture (listen to)	1.7
Downhill: 5-10% (2.5 mph)	3.6-3.5	Conversing	1.8
15-20% (2.5 mph)	3.7-4.3	Personal toilet	2.0
Hiking: 40 lb pack (3.0 mph)	6.8	Sitting, writing	2.6

Running:		Standing, light activity	2.6
12-min mile (5 mph)	10.0	Washing and dressing	2.6
8-min mile (7.5 mph)	15.0	Washing and shaving	2.6
6-min mile (10 mph)	20.0	Driving a car	2.8
5-min mile (12 mph)	25.0	Washing clothes	3.1
Mopping floors	4.9	Walking indoors	3.1
Repaving roads	5.0	Shining shoes	3.2
Gardening, weeding	5.6	Making bed	3.4
Stacking lumber	5.8	Dressing	3.4
Chain saw	6.2	Showering	3.4
Stone, masonry	6.3	Driving a motorcycle	3.4
Pick-and-shovel work	6.7	Metal working	3.5
Farming, haying, plowing with horse	6.7	House painting	3.5
Shoveling (miners)	6.8	Cleaning windows	3.7
Walking downstairs	7.1	Carpentry	3.8
Chopping wood	7.5	Farming chores	3.8
Crosscut saw	7.5-10.5	Sweeping floors	3.9
Tree felling (axe)	8.4-12.7	Plastering walls	4.1
Gardening, digging	8.6	Truck and automobile repair	4.2
Walking upstairs	10.0-18.0	Ironing clothes	4.2
Pool or billiards	1.8	Farming, planting, hoeing, raking	4.7
Canoeing: 2.5 mph-4.0 mph	3.0-7.0	Mixing cement	4.7
Volleyball: recreational-competitive	3.5-8.0		

Appendix 2: Activities and Associated Kilocalorie per Minute Expenditure (Marz, 1999)

CHAPTER THIRTEEN

Metabolism
Natural Nutrients vs. Stimulants
Andy Nelson, DC

Metabolism -- Natural Nutrients vs. Stimulants
By Andy Nelson, D.C.

When you attempt to diet, your body works against you by slowing down your metabolism. This occurs because our bodies are naturally programmed to store food for times of famine. Unfortunately, chronic dieters program their bodies for a new type of famine -- the next diet they go on! Many attempt to use chemical and herbal stimulants to overcome nature's famine response. These stimulants put undue stress on, and ultimately fatigue, the body. Learn how to triumph over the famine response with health-giving nutrients, balanced eating and moderate exercise.

A Novel Discovery with an Unexpected Twist

Anyone who knows a Chiropractor will tell you that they are always searching for some new discovery or scientific breakthrough to cure the world. In nine years of practice, I have attended countless seminars and paid over six figures looking for that better technique or the newest advancement in nutrition. In my search for new and better ways to address what we encounter on a daily basis; arthritis, the most common of all diseases [degenerative joint disease, also known as osteoarthritis], I discovered a new topical cream called EFAC (Esterified Fatty Acid Complex).

EFAC is an anti-inflammatory cellular lubricant that is clinically proven to be three times more effective than Glucosamine for joint pain so I had to try it. I have been using EFAC both as an oral softgel supplement, and a topical cream for several months now with excellent results. As a HealthSource clinic involved in weight loss, I also discovered another application for EFAC when incorporated into another solution for weight loss. Little did I know that I had happened upon a chiropractic coup d'etat! A revolutionary combination supplement for the relief of inflammation, joint pain and fat loss all at the same time!

It Just Gets Better

What if you could reduce stored fat, convert it into energy, preserve lean muscle and trim your waist all at the same time? What if a natural non-stimulant nutrient could help solve a host of diseases that are plaguing our society, including metabolic syndrome, a precursor to Non-Insulin Dependent Diabetes Mellitus (NIDDM), with no side effects. Metabolic syndrome is comprised of several metabolic components such as abdominal obesity, increased insulin in the blood stream, impaired glucose tolerance (sugar handling), high fasting blood glucose, high triglycerides, low HDL (good) cholesterol and hypertension (high blood pressure). It does all this by lowering leptin[1]...

Leptinology 101

Weight regulation is affected by leptin, which is a hormone produced in our adipose tissue (fat cells). Body fat was found to act as an endocrine gland (produces hormones) after very slim, young female athletes were found to have delays of the onset of their menstrual periods. It was discovered that the fat cells are a source of estrogen. Being very slim, the young athletes produced less estrogen, and hence their cycles were delayed. The effects of leptin on our health have been revealed after years of research.[2]

Leptin is now known to help regulate the storage of body fat. Leptin also affects our sense of fullness, blood sugar and our metabolism.[3] Attempts by scientists to lower leptin levels had been unsuccessful until researchers from the University of Minnesota were awarded a U.S. patent in May, 2005. The patent potentially represents one of the biggest breakthroughs in weight management. The patent was awarded because the researchers were able to prove that body fat and/or leptin levels could both be lowered using plant extracts.

These plant extracts are proprietary high viscosity polysaccharides which are a safe and natural blend of non-nutritive, plant-based, water soluble, non-starch, edible fiber. EFAC is added to these plant extracts to take advantage of the anti-inflammatory properties found in the compound. Inflammation can impact several areas of our health from arthritis to heart disease – even the process of aging. Research has proven that inflammation and pain almost always co-exist.

Inflammation and acidity almost always co-exist as in the case of a diet heavily weighted in animal products that promote a low acidic pH, whereas an alkaline environment is anti-inflammatory in nature, such as found in a plant-based diet with a high alkaline or basic pH. Inflammation is considered by leading scientists to be responsible for a number of metabolic problems which result in unwanted weight gain and obesity. Low grade, internal, invisible inflammation along with high leptin levels is at the very basis of excess body fat and the inability to lose excess or unwanted fat.

Is There Research to Support These Claims?

A well designed and highly controlled clinical trial was conducted by the University of Connecticut[3] to determine just how much impact high viscosity polysaccharides and esterified fatty acids would have. Women were placed in pairs for the duration of the trial, with one receiving the placebo and the other used the supplement. All women in the trial consulted weekly with a registered dietician. The women took part in an 8 week exercise program, cycling, walking or jogging

4 or 5 times a week. To ensure the women exercised similar amounts (therefore burning off a similar amount of calories) the researchers had the pairs exercise together.

The results were quite dramatic. All the women lost weight, as would be expected after taking part in this type of an exercise program. The amount and type of weight lost was very revealing. On placebo, the women lost on average 11.9 lbs, whereas the women on the supplement lost 20.2 lbs. The addition of the supplement enhanced the total weight loss by a remarkable 70%.

Even more impressive was the type of weight lost, as the supplement group of women had their percentage of body fat decrease by 7.4 points (43.6% to 36.2%) versus 3.4 points (44.3% to 40.9%) for the placebo group. The supplement group of women clearly lost more weight and the weight was primarily fat. The following data supports a preponderance of research and development into the combination of proprietary high viscosity polysaccharides and esterified fatty acid complex:

* Assists in promoting a lower percentage of body fat (Supported by US Patent 6,899,892 and references 1, 2, 3 and 4).
* Promotes the reduction of stored fat by increasing fatty acid utilization in the fat cell (Supported by references 4 and 5).
* Promotes the reduction of fat and an enhanced muscle to fat ratio (Supported by references 1, 2, 3 and 4).
* Promotes the regulation of energy balance allowing for improved mental energy (Supported by references 6 and 7).

References

1. Eikelis N and Esler M. The neurobiology of human obesity. Exp Physiol. 2005; (90)5: 673 – 682.
2. Drevon CA. Fatty acids and expression of adipokines. Bichimica et Biophysica Acta 2005, 1740: 287-292.
3. Meier U, Gressner AM. Endocrine regulation of energy metabolism: Review of pathobiochemical and clinical chemical aspects of leptin, ghrelin, adiponectin and resistin. Clin Chemistry 2004, 50(9): 1511-1525.
4. Cohen P, Miyazaki M, Socci ND, Hagge-Greenberg A, Liedtke W, Soukas AA, Sharma R, Hudgins LC, Ntambi JM, Friedman JM. Role for stearoyl-CoA desaturase-1 in leptin-mediated weight loss. Science. 2002 12; 297(5579):240-3.
5. Cohen P, Friedman JM. Leptin and the control of metabolism: role for stearoyl-CoA desaturase-1 (SCD-1). J Nutr. 2004 Sep; 134(9):2455S-2463S.
6. Greenwood CE, Winocur G. High-fat diets, insulin resistance and declining cognitive function. Neurobiol Aging. 2005 Oct 27.
7. Elias MF, Elias PK, Sullivan LM, Wolf PA, D'Agostino RB. Obesity, diabetes and cognitive deficit: The Framingham Heart Study. Neurobiol Aging. 2005 Oct 10.

A New Approach to Healthy Weight Loss - Lowering Leptin

A relatively new diet industry has sprung up called "Leptin Diets." In the early 1980's a hormone called leptin was discovered as the body's regulator of fat storage. Researchers found that the higher the leptin levels the greater the storage of fat.[4] Correspondingly, if leptin levels can be lowered, then the body is signaled to release stored and dietary fat for other purposes, most predominately as energy.

In a scientific setting, researchers have attempted to lower leptin. Continuous and excessive levels of exercise <u>do not</u> lower leptin levels. A low fat diet <u>does not</u> lower leptin. In fact, many of the fat free cookies, cakes, corn chips, etc. actually cause leptin levels to rise, thereby modifying the body to being even more efficient at storing fat.

Diets <u>do not</u> lower leptin. In fact, very low calorie diets (VLCD) place the body in a moderate mode of starvation causing the body to become more efficient at storing fat. Appetite suppressants or calorie restricted diets alone may offer short term "weight loss" (water and muscle), and more weight gain (fat) in the future. Weight loss is predominantly water and lean muscle loss. Your fat to muscle ratio rises and you have set-up your body to become very efficient at storing fat.

Appetite suppressants <u>do not</u> work in the long term because once again your body goes into a mode of starvation and is positioned to become proficient at storing fat. There exists a genetic predisposition to efficiently store fat for survival in the short term, particularly as we age. The problem is that leptin levels rise as we age, which works for the short term survival for people during famines or shortages of food supplies. However, high leptin levels are a primary contributor to heart disease, diabetes and have an amazingly correlative relationship to the storage of fat around the waist for men; waist, hips and thighs for women.

The lowering of leptin levels provides an entirely new approach to weight loss. Leptin also affects satiation (feeling full), glycemic control and metabolism. Because of the connection between leptin levels and body fat, there were many attempts by scientists to lower leptin levels. The safety profile of these leptin lowering plant extracts are in stark contrast to stimulants such as ephedra or caffeine containing plants.

For Every Action, There Is an Opposite and Equal Reaction

I had a patient that told me a sad tale of his trip to Mexico on vacation with his girlfriend and his son. On their way home, he was tired and consumed an energy drink to stay awake while he drove. According to my patient's account, the energy drink gave him a short term boost of alertness, and then he crashed, literally! He had fallen asleep because of the false security that the energy drink's initial wave of stimulation gave, only to succumb to his very real need for sleep. He fell asleep at the wheel and the crash was fatal to his girlfriend. His son had minor injuries and my patient had fractured his spine. What a tragedy!

The average 8-ounce energy drink contains around 80 mg of caffeine, with more and more brands appearing with even more caffeine. People use energy drinks for desired effects of increased energy and mental alertness, similar to the use of stimulants in weight loss supplements. However, there are some negative side effects that include nervousness, irritability, sleeplessness, increased urination, abnormal heart rhythms, decreased bone density, and stomach upset.

Stimulants such as caffeine, ephedrine and nicotine have not been clinically proven to increase metabolic rates. It may be that they stimulate a person to simply be more active (sometimes agitated or jittery), which then burns more calories. Some of these products can be harmful and are not recommended.

Another little known fact is that stimulants put undue stress on the adrenal gland due to an autonomic response of sympathetic (fight or flight) dominance that triggers a cascade of other hormonal reactions that often affect the endocrine (glandular) system's negative feedback loop. Repeated insults to this negative feedback loop will often cause adrenal fatigue and result in under active thyroid function which lowers your metabolism. What at first over stimulated your body, now ends up fatiguing your body, and you are left feeling tired and lethargic, lacking the very energy you were at first seeking.

In the chiropractic paradigm, Newton's third law of motion equally applies to natural medicine as well as pharmaceutical medicine. His posit was that "for every action, there is an equal and opposite reaction." This explains perfectly why most all medications have adverse reactions or complications. The intelligence of the body strives for homeostasis (same state) or balance, so that medications disturb that balance and cause reactions within the body. Hippocrates said it best as he is quoted, "Let foods be your medicine." My favorite supplements are whole food based, which include all the synergistic co-factors and trace elements needed for your body to truly assimilate these nutrients.

Eat GRAS!

No, this isn't a misspelling. GRAS stands for Generally Regarded As Safe. This is the U.S. government's rating for food additives that may serve as a best measure of safety. The high viscosity polysaccharide plant extracts I have mentioned have a GRAS rating, and many other nutritional supplements are generally regarded as safe, with no known adverse effects.

Now, foods do come in pill form, so don't throw the baby out with the bathwater just because something comes in a pill form. There are some pretty incredible natural botanicals such as Acai, Mangosteen, Resveratrol, forskolin, Wakame Seaweed, herbal detox cleanses and the list goes on. That list can be lengthy, confusing and expensive, so for our purposes, I have focused on just a few. Green tea drinkers were shown to burn an extra 70 calories per day in a recent study. Researchers believe the increase is caused by antioxidants known as catechin polyphenols, particularly epigallocatechin gallate (EGCG). Green tea polyphenols are known to promote weight loss as an extract without the properties of caffeine by increasing the metabolism of fats in the liver (thermogenic effect) and inhibiting lipase (fat absorption enzyme) in the digestive tract.. Recent high-quality study[5] demonstrated that green tea can reduce body weight in obese persons by increasing energy expenditure and fat oxidation. The results of new Japanese study[6] also confirm fat-burning properties of green tea. Researches found that continuous ingestion of a green tea extract high in catechins led to a reduction in body fat, systolic blood pressure, and LDL cholesterol.

Survival of the Fittest, not the Fattest

Ancestral survival mechanisms have changed with the abundance of calorie-rich food.

Genetically speaking, our body is predisposed to be very efficient at storing fat for survival purposes. With the access to caloric dense foods and modern lifestyle, our body easily stores excess energy intake as fat. The regulation of body fat storage includes the integration of hormonal action. Scientists have recently discovered that two key hormones play a dominant role in the storage of fat, particularly around the waistline. The leptin hormone is a strong signal for regulating fat storage in adipocytes, or fat cells. It has been confirmed in a number of clinical trials that as leptin increases there is a corresponding increase in fat storage. Additionally, the adiponectin hormone plays a key role in signaling the body to reduce muscle and also increase fat as we age. If it was possible to balance these hormones, a more enhanced body composition would take place by accelerating the reduction of fat and increasing lean muscle. The result would be an improved fat to muscle ratio for a more youthful body.

An interesting anecdotal story is the account of one of the researchers from the University of Minnesota studying high viscosity polysaccharides and esterified fatty acid complex. A 55-year man of normal weight who had always been athletic used the supplement for one year. Despite being athletic, he retained belly fat as many of us do. However, for the first time in his life, he started to develop a six-pack in his abdominal region. His goal was not to lose weight, and his total weight loss was only 10 lbs., but he lost his cravings for sugar and increased his fat to muscle ratio which resulted in improved muscle definition.

How to Make This Discovery Work for You

High viscosity polysaccharides and esterified fatty acids have been shown to enhance your efforts to lose fat, and thus effectively lose weight. How fast it works largely depends on your efforts. If you are performing aerobic exercise regularly you can expect better and faster results, which occurred quite impressively in the 8 week clinical trial. It has not been tested without increased physical activity. Judging by anecdotal reports in which people's level of physical activity did not change, it will likely help to increase fat loss and reduce food cravings, but that it will take a number of months to start to do so.

In addition, feedback to date has been that the impact is greater when taken consistently. Feedback regarding inconsistent use (for example, take it for a few weeks and then stop and restart a few weeks later) has been that the reduction of weight and regulation of sugar cravings takes a very long time.

Make fat loss your goal, not weight loss

It is important to remember that all weight loss is not equal. Fat loss has a far greater positive health impact than general weight loss that consists of a combination of fat, muscle and water weight. Losing weight causes your metabolic rate (the rate at which you burn fat) to come to a complete halt. Losing fat and increasing lean muscle tissue sends your metabolic rate through the roof which is the key to staying permanently thin.

The bottom line is that fat loss increases your metabolism, whereas muscle loss decreases your metabolism. For long-term weight management, the higher your metabolism, the easier it is to control your weight. In addition, the supplement group experienced other important health benefits, as their leptin and insulin levels were both lowered.

When it comes to muscle loss, as happens with very low calorie diets, our metabolism is lowered. This is because our muscles use a lot of energy and therefore when you lose muscle, you then require fewer calories to function, or in other words your metabolic rate is reduced. This is precisely the risk of very low calorie diets, as the body burns muscle tissue to make up for the deficit in calories consumed. In essence our body uses our muscles for food.

A lowered metabolism makes effective long-term weight management more difficult. Regretfully, repeated crash dieting with very low calories being consumed, is believed to result in the up and down or "Yo-Yo" diets, which tend to cause weight to increase over time.

On the other hand fat loss can increase our metabolism. This is because our metabolism is determined by the usage of energy by the various body tissues. Fat and muscle are the two prime tissues upon which our metabolism is based, and therefore our metabolism is largely determined by a ratio of these two tissues. The greatest positive impact on metabolism occurs when we lose fat and at the same time build muscle by exercising. For continued long-term success of weight management, the key therefore becomes fat loss and the avoidance of muscle loss.

Customize Calculate Your Calories to Churn and Burn

Regardless of what nutritional approach you take, there is no getting away with losing fat for good without lowering calories and exercising. Here's the simplest and most accurate method that I have found for calculating the minimum amount of calories your body needs at rest, to stay alive and maintain your current body weight. This is called your Basal Metabolic Rate (BMR) or Resting Energy Expenditure (REE). We will use the Mifflin equation, published in the February 1990 issue of the American Journal of Clinical Nutrition:

Mifflin Equation

<u>Men:</u> BMR = [9.99 x (wt. in lbs./2.2)] + [6.25 x (ht. in in. x 2.54)] − [4.92 x age] + 5

<u>Women:</u> BMR = [9.99 x (wt. in lbs./2.2)] + [6.25 x (ht. in in. x 2.54)] − [4.92 x age) − 161

Remember the commutative property from High School. Work out the parentheses first, then the brackets, and work from left to right. The sum of this formula is called your Total Daily Energy Expenditure (TDEE) measured in kCal/day.

To determine your total daily calorie needs, the BMR is multiplied by the appropriate activity factor, as follows:

- 1.200 = sedentary (little or no exercise)
- 1.375 = lightly active (light exercise/sports 1-3 days/week)
- 1.550 = moderately active (moderate exercise/sports 3-5 days/week)
- 1.725 = very active (hard exercise/sports 6-7 days a week)
- 1.900 = extra active (very hard exercise/sports and physical job)

Example: 46 year old female, 5'-6" tall (66"), 186 lbs., lightly active, BMI* = 30 (Obese)

Body Mass Index of 24 is ideal. For this person, her goal weight would be 148 lbs. The Institute of Medicine has stated that the "normal" BMI range is from 18.5 to 24.9.

Plugging the numbers into the Mifflin formula for women, and factor in the activity level as follows:

[9.99 x (84.55)] + [6.25 x (167.64)] − [226.32] − 161   x Activity Factor = TDEE = 844.65   +   1047.75   − 226.32 − 161 = **1,505 x 1.375 = 2,069 kcal/day**

Now, let's reduce those calories in order to lose weight, also called caloric deficit. This creates a negative energy balance, when expenditure (metabolic rate) is greater than consumption. To create a calorie deficit you want to: 1) eat fewer calories than you consume, or 2) add more activity to burn more calories, or 3) do both; eat fewer calories and add exercises to help you lose weight. The most common guideline for calorie deficits for fat loss is to reduce your calories by at least 500, but not more than 1000 calories below your TDEE, for an average 1 -2 pounds lost per week.

The American College of Sports Medicine (ACSM) recommends that calorie levels never drop below 1200 calories per day for women or 1800 per day for men. Reducing calories by 15-20% below TDEE is a good place to start. A larger deficit may be necessary in some cases, but the best approach would be to keep the calorie deficit through diet small while increasing activity level.

Putting it All Together
- 5 Ways to Boost Your Metabolism

1. Increase muscle mass through strength training 3-4 times per week, and aerobic exercise 3 days per week.
2. Regulate insulin levels by dividing your daily calorie consumption into 6 small meals or snacks, and eat protein rich foods, on average 70-90 grams per day. Also, don't skip meals or decrease calories too drastically!
3. Increase movement in your daily routine by walking the dog or taking the stairs. You'll burn extra calories by practicing the chiropractic credo: "Motion is life."
4. Get adequate sleep. Too little will decrease your metabolism.
5. Lower leptin levels with proven, natural stimulant-free supplements such as high viscosity polysaccharides, and reduce inflammation with esterified fatty acid complex. Take green tea extract. Alkalize your body with non-inflammatory foods by eating 5-9 servings of fresh fruits and vegetables daily. Take fish oil and use olive oils frequently. Avoid stimulants and those things that are not GRAS.

Lastly, use a system and follow a plan with goals set forth under the direction of a qualified doctor. Use foods that have known quantities of caloric intake for optimal control and measurable results. Make fat loss your goal, and get that metabolism going.

[1] Topping, D.L. et al., "A Viscous Fibre (Methylcellulose) Lowers Blood Glucose and Plasma Triglycerols and Increases Liver Glycogen Independently of Volatile Fatty Acid Production...," British Journal of Nutrition (1988), 59, 21-30 (March 10, 1987)

[2] Fried et al., Elevation in Serum Leptin Levels in Obesity, J. Nutr. (2000) 3127S-3131S

[3] Levin et al., "Leptin is a Satiety Factor and a Regulator of Metabolism," 1996 Proc. Natl. Acad. Sci. USA 93:1726-1730

[4] Fragala MS, et al., "Influences of a Dietary Supplement in Combination with an Exercise and Diet Regimen on Adipocytokines and Adiposity in Women Who Are Overweight. Eur. J Appl. Physiol. 2009 Mar;105(5):665-72. Epub 2008 Dec 2.

[5] Auvichayapat Pet al., "Effectiveness of green tea on weight reduction in obese." Thais: A randomized, controlled trial. Physiol. Behav. 2007 Oct 18

[6] Nagao T, Hase T, Tokimitsu I. "A Green Tea Extract High in Catechins Reduces Body Fat and Cardiovascular Risks in Humans." Obesity (Silver Spring). 2007 Jun;15(6):1473-83.

"Guts are important. Your guts are what digest things. But it is your brains that tell you which things to swallow and which not to swallow."
Austin Dacey

Chapter Fourteen

Breaking Through Plateaus
By Jim Hoven, DC

Breaking Through Plateaus
By Jim Hoven, DC

Your weight loss has been progressing nicely. The program you've dedicated yourself to has shown definite results not only in weight loss, but in a loss of inches and in body fat as well. Your morale is high as the momentum of your progress keeps you going. Then suddenly it happens, the one thing that everyone engaged in a serious weight loss program dreads but understands as inevitable... the PLATEAU.

The Plateau is indeed the most frustrating and nerve-racking part of any weight loss program, and it is often at this point in the weight loss process where doubt creeps in to the mind and can literally send both you and your entire program into a tailspin. Because the Plateau can represent a crossroads for future success in weight loss, it's critically important to understand the nature of plateaus, why they occur, and what to do about them in order to get through them as quickly as possible, not only physically, but mentally and emotionally as well.

The word plateau can be defined as:
plateau [plat-oh, -ohs]
Noun a relatively long period of stability:
Verb to remain stable for a long period [French]
Collins Essential English Dictionary

Understanding Plateaus in Weight Loss

When we examine the definition of the word itself, a plateau is a fairly benign and neutral state. It is in looking

Chapter 14 | Breaking Through Plateaus: Understanding Plateaus in Weight Loss

at this definition that we can relax and find some peace with the experience of the Plateau . In fact, if you think about it, all things in life work in a cyclical basis and as such will have a stage of plateau within them. For example, there comes a point in every relationship between two people where growth has occurred and they know each other fairly well. Once the relationship achieves a level of familiarity, things become stationary for a period of time until a new stimulus is introduced into the relationship causing it to move forward at a deeper or more intense level.

The same could be said of the learning process. If you were studying any subject, you would get to a point where you were reasonably proficient in that topic and could operate in an effective mode for an extended period of time. However, for you to become an expert in that subject, you would need to increase your knowledge base and combine it with the experience of what you learned in the past in order to move to a new level of expertise.

One more example on plateaus that relates to each and every one of us revolves around our job, occupation, or profession. Think back to a time when you were a learning a new job or a new duty at your place of work. You spent hours asking questions, meeting with people, pouring over manuals and digging into your assignments with gusto in order to get to a level of proficiency at that job, task, or duty. Your skill set grew to the point where you were able to perform the required actions with a fairly low level of effort. It is at that moment in time when you arrived at a plateau. If you did nothing further from that point, the likelihood of you finding continued growth, success, and motivation in that job or even in that career field would also plateau, and would probably result in you not progressing forward in that job, that company, or in that career.

How Learning From the Past Creates Success In The Future

The reason I pointed out different types of plateaus that commonly occur throughout life was so that you might relate to one or more of them and then fully realize that not only have you seen plateaus in other areas of your life before, but you have overcome them as well!

Now that we've identified the fact that plateaus occur throughout our lives, the next logical question is... Why do we have to experience plateaus? The answer is really very simple and can be summarized in one word, EFFICIENCY!!! Everything in the universe wants to work at the most efficient level possible. That means getting the best results from the least amount of work.

You can see this concept in action everywhere throughout nature. Plants grow the most when conditions such as temperature and moisture are optimal for growth, animals search for food during times when food is most likely to be found as well as when their bodies have the greatest energy to find it, and as water flows downhill it always takes the path of least resistance. Just as plants, animals, and water utilize the principle of efficiency, our bodies do too!

When you began your weight loss program, you set up a specific plan with respect to the amount of calories you would take in every day, the sources from which you would obtain those calories, and the amount of exercise that you would perform during a given day or week. Once you began that program, your body immediately went into action based upon the new "stresses" that you were putting upon it. It knew that because you were taking in fewer calories than it needed to adapt, and because you began walking, your muscular system and your cardiovascular system had to adapt. The net result of all this adapting was a loss in weight and inches.

Over time (a period of weeks or months), your body's efficiency improved and it became used to consuming fewer calories for fuel. It also became used to the amount and type of exercise that you were doing. The result of the increase in efficiency was the ability for your body to perform all of its daily functions under the new conditions that you placed upon it with less effort than before.

The good news is that your body is working exactly as it was designed to. Imagine yourself living in conditions where food was scarce and where you had to exert a high level of energy in order to find the things you needed to survive(like food , water and shelter). You want your body to be able to deal with adverse conditions if you had to go extended periods of time between meals, or if you had to cross rivers or climb mountains in order to find shelter. While your body's ability to be efficient is excellent in a survival situation, it isn't so good for ongoing weight loss.

What Does the Body's Basal Metabolic Rate Have To Do With Weight?

There are a couple of reasons why the body's efficiency slows down or even stops weight loss. The first has to do with the body's Basal Metabolic Rate (BMR). The BMR is essentially a measurement of how well your body burns calories. The higher your BMR, the more calories you burn throughout your day. There are several factors that influence your BMR including your body weight, the number of calories you take in on a daily basis, and the amount of calories you burn. As you begin to lose weight, your BMR decreases!

Because you are lighter, your body does not have to work as hard to sustain its systems and activities. This is the perfect example of your body being efficient. For continued weight loss to occur, you must find a way to keep your body's BMR up and running at a high rate. The second reason has to do with calorie intake. When you begin to cut your calories, your weight drops.

After a period of time, the body weight will drop to a level where the number of calories required to support it becomes less than what you are taking in. For example, if you were eating 3000 calories per day prior to beginning your weight loss program, and reduced your caloric intake to 2000 calories per day, you would begin to lose weight in a very short time.

At a certain point however, you would find a level where the 2000 calories you were taking in every day would be more than what the body needed to support continued weight loss. At that point in time, calories would need to be restricted further or exercise would need to be increased in order to get continued weight loss.

CHAPTER 14 | BREAKING THROUGH PLATEAUS:
UNDERSTANDING PLATEAUS IN WEIGHT LOSS

The Top Tips To Accelerate Your Weight Loss Breakthrough

So, while the principle of efficiency is critical for our ability to survive, it is also the biggest reason why you have hit the Plateau in your weight loss efforts, and it must be addressed in three areas if you are to move past the Plateau and onto further weight-loss success.

1. Nutrition: As mentioned previously, when a weight-loss plateau is reached, it is often due to the fact that the calorie requirements of your new body weight are less than that of what you are taking in. It's important to examine the amount of calories required for you to get to your next body weight goal and then compare that to the amount of calories that you are actually taking in. A good rule of thumb is to take your goal weight and multiply it by a factor of 10 to get a basic number of calories that you should be ingesting on a daily basis. For example, if you are at 160 pounds and wanted to weigh 150 pounds, a good starting point would be for you to take in 1500 calories per day (150x10).

There are multiple sites located on the Internet where you can calculate the approximate number of calories required for daily consumption. Keep in mind when using these web based programs, that they are only averages, and that you must use your best judgment based on the results that you are seeing as to whether this number is accurate for you or not. To find a program on the web, simply go to an Internet search engine and type in Daily Caloric Intake Calculator.

With respect to calories, another important exercise is to carefully examine the exact amount and types of calories that you are taking in.

It's not uncommon for people to think they are taking in a certain number of calories but, upon a thorough inspection, realized that they were actually ingesting quite a bit more than what they had thought. This usually occurs due to the addition of specific things into the diet like dressings for salads and condiments such as ketchup, mustard, mayonnaise, steak sauce, etc. that are not considered when doing calorie calculations.

Another insidious source of calorie pileup comes from unchecked snacking. A few chips here, a handful of candy there, a small soda or fruit juice all add up to what can be a surprisingly high number of calories. It is possible to be incredibly accurate with respect to the number of calories taken in on a daily basis. The Internet has made it possible to track every item imaginable with respect to calorie content, as well as the amount of protein, carbohydrates, fats, vitamins and minerals present in each and every food.

To find one of these sites, simply do a search for Calorie Counter on the Internet and choose one that is easy for you to navigate. It should be noted here that to get completely accurate results, you must put in completely accurate data. These sites allow for customization of individual items. Specifically, you can enter the nutritional facts including calories, fat, cholesterol, protein, carbohydrates, etc. for any item not listed on the website. Entering a food one time puts it into the system and keeps it there for you to use in your calculations from there forward. A little work on the front end, or as you go through your daily routine will allow you to know within seconds the exact number and type of calories that you've been taking in. This is an unbelievably valuable tool for consistent weight loss.

2. Exercise: Weight loss is the net effect between calories taken in and calories burned or expended. We've already talked about the number of calories taken in and how that affects your BMR. It is exercise that creates the other half of the equation. Many people do little to no exercise when starting a weight-loss program. They typically avoid exercise because their bodies have multiple aches and pains making exercise uncomfortable or even painful, they are unsure about what exercises are best, or they are self-conscious about their appearance and what others might be thinking or saying about them.

If you've experienced a plateau in your weight loss efforts and you have not yet incorporated an exercise program, this may very well be the ticket to getting you off of your plateau. There are two major forms of exercise involved in optimal weight loss. The first is cardiovascular training. Cardiovascular training is one way to keep the BMR elevated even after your weight loss has resulted in a decreased caloric requirement for basic body function.

If you remember from earlier in the chapter, as body weight drops, so does BMR. Regular cardiovascular exercise is a great way to keep the BMR working as efficiently as possible and promoting continued weight loss. The second primary form of exercise comes in the form of resistance training. Most people think of this as weight training, which if you've never performed this type of exercise in the past, can be intimidating. The key concept with resistance training is that it doesn't have to be with weights. Often, low-tech devices such as bands, tubes, and handles can be used with great effectiveness. Programs can be designed with the use of these very simple, low-tech items to be done at home in a combination with simple body movements requiring no extra weight whatsoever.

More will be spoken about the subject of exercise later in this book. In the event that you have been performing a regular exercise routine and have hit a plateau, there is one critical yet simple concept that will combat that dreaded principle of efficiency and get you moving forward again…

3.   Change your routine!! Alter the exercises that you are doing. For example, if you have been performing the same lifts and cardio training for your upper and your lower body over the last several weeks to months, it's time to shake things up. Find other movements that work the same muscles in a different way. Change the weight you are using on your workouts. Change the tempo at which you exercise (decrease rest time between sets, increase the number of sets or reps, or try going from a slow, steady speed to a more high-intensity interval training program). If you're not sure how to do any of these things, there are a myriad of books and Internet articles on the subject, or you can hire a personal trainer to show you a group of exercises that you can use to achieve the next level of training and the next level of results. Remember, you've got to keep the body guessing when it comes to exercise. The more your body becomes familiar with a single routine, the more efficient it becomes, and the less weight you lose. It's a great idea to make some kind of change to your exercise routine every 4 to 6 weeks to keep things new, fresh, and effective.

4.   Mental and emotional focus: The longer a plateau lasts, the more you want to go crazy. Extended plateaus can lead to more than just a lack of progress; they can lead to self doubt, the temptation to quit, and in some cases even clinical depression. Because of the potential disastrous consequences of extended plateaus, it is critical to develop a set of skills on how to mentally and emotionally handle plateaus as well as how to get through them.

When on a plateau, take a moment to look back from where it is that you've come. Whether you've lost five, 10, 20 pounds or more, you have done a great job! Oftentimes, seeing what you've accomplished can give you the sense of pride and accomplishment as well as the stamina to continue onward. You must take the time to celebrate your accomplishments and your victories!

Do not tie your worthiness as a human being to the amount of weight you lose. You are a wonderful and amazing person. You were created that way! The journey you began when you started the weight loss process was not just about a number (the pounds you were going to lose), but about how you would change your level of health for the remainder of your life and who you would become as a person in the process. Remembering the bigger picture of who you are while you are undergoing this transformation is the best way to fight the temptation of unworthiness that a plateau often generates. Once you have overcome the emotional negativity associated with a plateau, and you realize that you are on a path that is destined for success, you need to incorporate the principle of Mental Toughness. Becoming mentally tough results in the development of several important characteristics including persistence and determination.

Characteristics such as these lead to success in every area of life and are especially important in the face of both difficulty and adversity. Being mentally tough when facing a weight-loss plateau will result in an attitude of dogged determination that you will eventually succeed, and that you will find a way. It is this attitude that leads to an increase in your creative ability to see options and opportunities for moving forward in your program. To get off of a weight-loss plateau, or any plateau for that matter, these are the characteristics that lead to success. You can find much more information on the emotional components of weight-loss in chapter 10 of this book written by Dr. Patrick Porter.

Plateaus are a natural part of life, as well as a natural part of any significant weight loss program. By understanding how to manipulate the variables of calories, exercise, and mental outlook you can get off of the plateau and onto continued weight loss success.

"In order to succeed, your desire for success should be greater than your fear of failure. "
Bill Cosby

CHAPTER FIFTEEN

EATING A BALANCED MEAL
Michele Askar, DC

EATING A BALANCED MEAL
Michele Askar, DC

What are you currently doing when preparing your meals?

How is that working for you? In this chapter, I will show you how to change your thought processes about food and how to create a balanced meal for optimum health.

Let me start off by saying you don't want to set yourself up for failure and you don't want to fall into the common misconception that you need to avoid your favorite foods to lose weight. This is just not the case. The sample meals I provide are easy to prepare and will give your body the nutrients and energy it needs. I have also included a meal log to prepare your meals in advance in order to assist you in eating balanced meals with small snacks.

What are your goals?

Once you have decided to eat better because you have identified the reason to change your habits, the next question you must answer is, what are your top five most important goals you need to accomplish to be pleased with your progress that will keep you on track with your program of exercising and eating better? The idea of eating a balanced meal is to ingest the proper amount of calories based upon your age, height, and weight, using the BMI calculator.

So you may be asking yourself what is the best way for me?

There are some key factors that will assist you in achieving your goal. First you need to know the basics of losing weight as discussed in Chapter 10 by changing your beliefs. Secondly, you must learn to exercise and eat balanced meals, and lastly, you must create self-motivation.

After years of my own experience in dieting and being an obsess teenager, I realized that eating balanced meals was a key component to any weight loss program that I tried and that it can also be confusing on how and where to start. So I have created a meal log and included some tasty recipes to get you started.

Please remember that one of the most beautiful things about us being human beings is our ability to adapt and evolve. We have the opportunity to re-design ourselves, if we chose to, and know how to. (As Dr. Porter taught in Chapter 10.)

As the old adage goes, "you are what you eat and unfortunately most people don't understand it.

What I have observed is that most people have no clue what they are doing to themselves by the foods they choose to eat. Nor do they realize how good they can feel or how good they can look by making better food choices.

So let me teach you a better method for creating a balance meal.

Listed below are some examples of Nutrient Rich Foods:

Tuna	*Whole Wheat Bread*	*Broccoli*
Chicken	*Apples*	*Onions*
Lean Ham	*Oranges*	*Mushrooms*
Lean Ground Turkey	*Strawberries*	*Lettuce*
Salmon	*Melons*	*Tomatoes*
Crab	*Pasta*	*Spinach*
Chicken Breast	*Baked Potato*	*Cucumber*
Turkey Breast	*Oatmeal*	*Carrots*
Low-Fat Cottage Cheese	*Steamed Brown Rice*	*Green Beans*
Egg Whites	*Steamed Wild Rice*	*Celery*

The idea is to choose one item from each column to create a balanced meal. For example, salmon, baked potato, and green beans. I'll show you other examples later in this chapter.

What is the hidden secret to success?

Another thing you can do to guarantee your success in creating a balanced meal is make sure the foods in your refrigerator, freezers and cabinets are stocked with the right foods to re-design yourself. So make a list before you go to the grocery store, only stocking up on quality foods such as proteins, carbohydrates and vegetables.

A lesson I learned a long time ago that I want to pass on to you is to allow yourself a cheat day. Eat whatever you want because I was told the psychological and physiological reasons behind that was that it helps convince the body that you are not starving it and you won't feel so constrained which allows

Chapter 15 | Eating a Balanced Meal

you to get back on track the next day. This little piece of info helped me to never fail at a weight loss goal because I never felt that I was deprived and we all want to win. You choose which day of the week is your free day and stick to that day remembering it can change. If a special event is coming up, you can adjust accordingly.

What follows are samples of a few meals that I have created with a guide to help you step by step to chart your meals so you can track where you are and where you are going. It will allow you the ability to modify your meals so you can continually reach your goals. Most importantly, it's about quality not quantity.

DATE:
PLANNED MEAL
BREAKFAST
SNACK
LUNCH
SNACK
DINNER
SNACK

BALANCED DIET MEALS FOR ONE WEEK

BREAKFAST

DAY ONE

1 Whole Egg or two egg whites
3 slices of turkey bacon
½ English muffin (multi-grain), no butter or spray butter

DAY TWO

¾ Cup Cereal, ½ Cup Skim Milk, ½ banana, or ½ cup blueberries (your choice)

DAY THREE

2 Whole eggs scrambled to make omelet with your choice of peppers, onions, tomatoes,

Add parsley or spice to your liking.

DAY FOUR

¾ cup low fat yogurt with ½ cup cereal mixed in or ¾ cup berries or fruit

DAY FIVE

Shake, 1 cup skim milk, 1 cup ice, 1 banana or ½ banana and ½ cup other fruit or no banana and 1 cup fruit and blend.

DAY SIX

Small Breakfast Sandwich – 1 slice multigrain toast cut in half, 1 egg fried w/spray butter, 1 slice of cheese or 2 slices of turkey or 1 slice of regular bacon.

BREAKFAST DRINKS

1 Cup Coffee, Skim Milk and 1 tsp Sugar OR if you have to ½ cup diluted juice with lots of water.

BALANCED DIET – LUNCH –SNACK

DAY ONE

Green salad (the more greens the lettuce the better (more nutrients)), toppings: mushrooms, peppers, onions, cucumbers, tomatoes, etc. Either 2 eggs whites, 3 oz. chicken, fresh tuna (no additives)

DAY TWO

1 Cup or ½ Cup Soup: vegetable, wedding, chick w/veggies, chicken noodle. Sprinkle cheese just enough to cover top. 5 or 6 croutons.

DAY THREE

3-6 Oz. of chicken breast, fish, or turkey breast. Small side salad –vinaigrette dressing, Italian low fat (check carbohydrates) dressing. (No croutons) 1 small potato (baked) or ½ potato.

DAY FOUR
Same meat as Day three, your choice of at least 1 cup to 1 ½ cups veggies preferable: sugar snap peas, regular peas, beans, or broccoli, ½ cup whole grain rice.

DAY FIVE
Make your own tuna salad (1 full cup) w/light mayo, and celery. On top of green lettuce and a few shavings of cheese. 5 to 6 croutons are allowed.

DAY SIX
1 Slice whole grain bread, top it with 2 slices low or no-fat ham or turkey breast, fresh tomatoes, lettuce. One tbsp of light mayo you can add pickles or onions.

DRINKS FOR LUNCH
Water, unsweetened peppermint tea w/lemon (Any herbal tea)

DINNER PLAN
DAY ONE
NOTE: You can mix the meat with ground turkey.
Hamburger (3-6 oz.) chooses the leanest meat available (93/7) - 7 percent fat. Use a grill or type of pan that allows the remaining fat to run off. No bun, 1 thin slice of cheese. Your choice of veggies to top. Ketchup and mustard are allowed. Half of a sweet potato and 1 cup of spinach or other green vegetable.

DAY TWO – Steak Stir Fry
Steak 3-6 oz. cut off fat before cooking. Grill it or use pan to prevent eating any remaining fat. Steam ¾ cup brown rice. Choose 4-5 veggies – sugar snap peas, broccoli, onion, zucchini, and fry in tsp butter or fat free spray butter. Cut steak into small bite size pieces. Mix steak rice and veggies together.

DAY THREE

Grilled chicken breast. Marinate chicken in fresh squeezed lemon juice, fresh basil, thyme, whatever spices you like, overnight. Grill chicken. One small baked potato or ½ big potato. 5-6 stalks of grilled asparagus.

DAY FOUR

Ham steak. Steam 1 precooked lean ham steak. 1 ½ cup steamed broccoli. ½ cup baked beans. Cut ham in half for 1 portion.

DAY FIVE

Shrimp Pasta – Using 1 tsp extra virgin olive oil in pan sauté 1 ¼ cup peeled shrimp with fresh lemon, your choice of spices. 1 ½ cup angel hair pasta. When shrimp is almost done, put 1 cup your choice of chopped vegetable.

DAY SIX

Cut 1 large chicken breast or 8 oz. into bite size squares, sauté in 1 tbsp extra virgin olive oil with 1 ¼ cup peeled eggplant (with or w/o seeds cut into squares) cut 2 fresh tomatoes and 1 ¼ cup squash add to chicken with ¼ cup jar sauce, mix together. Add seasonings of your choice. Makes 2 servings.

Always drink water or non caffeinated soda. No cocktails. Cocktails can add an additional 65-160 calories per drink.

HEALTHY SNACKS

Fresh fruit once a day for snack (preferably in AM)
Any fresh vegetables
Pretzels (a few a day)

DR. ASKAR'S WEIGHT LOSS TIPS

1. Set attainable goals.
2. Start your diet with a food journal and record everything you eat.
3. Drink six to eight glasses of water everyday.
4. Avoid eating with the TV on or in front of the TV. It tends to make you snack more heavily.
5. Weigh yourself once a week at the same time.
6. If you plateau @ a certain weight, don't panic. It's your body getting used to the new you. Drink more water, or reduce your calories.
7. Don't shop when you are hungry.
8. Don't deprive yourself. Acknowledge your cheat day.
9. Lose weight for yourself, not your spouse, mother or friends.
10. NEVER skip meals.
11. Try to avoid sugar. The more you have the more you crave.
12. Lose 2-5 lbs. more than your goal to give yourself room to fluctuate.
13. When eating out, eat your salad first to dull your appetite before the main course.
14. Skip the second glass of wine or cocktail before dinner, instead of skipping breakfast.
15. Go for a walk after you eat. It brings on *"exercise-induced postprandial thermogensis,"* which means the production of extra body heat created by exercising on a full stomach. The heat in a real sense melts body fat.

Recipes to design a balanced meal for you:

HONEY MUSTARD CHICKEN

- 2 tablespoons honey
- 1 tablespoon Dijon-style mustard
- 1 tablespoon lemon juice
- ½ teaspoon poppy seed
- ¼ teaspoon pepper
- 2 whole medium chicken breasts (about 1 ½ pounds total), skinned and halved lengthwise

- Add soy sauce, cilantro, tarragon
- In a small bowl combine honey, mustard, lemon juice, poppy seed, and pepper.
- Stir together well.
- Rinse chicken, pat dry.
- Place chicken bone side up, on the unheated rack of a broiler pan.
- Broil 4 to 5 inches from heat for 15 minutes.
- Turn. Continue broiling for 10 minutes.
- Brush with honey-mustard mixture.
- Broil about 5 minutes more or till tender and no longer pink.
- Makes 4 servings.

NUTRITION INFORMATION PER SERVING

168 calories, 1 g saturated fat, 1 g monounsaturated fat, 1 g polyunsaturated fat, 24 g protein, 9 g carbohydrate, 0 g dietary fiber, 65 mg cholesterol, 174 mg sodium, 210 mg potassium.

TURKEY-APPLE SAUSAGE

1   slightly beaten egg white
¼   cup soft bread crumbs
¼   cup finely chopped peeled apple
¼   teaspoon salt
¼   teaspoon ground sage
1/8 teaspoon pepper
½   pound ground raw turkey breast, lean ground raw turkey, or lean ground beef
Apple slices (optional)
Fresh sage leaves (optional)
Add onions (small)

In a medium mixing bowl combine egg white, bread crumbs, apple, salt, sage, and pepper. Add ground turkey or beef; mix well. Shape into eight small patties, about 2 ½ inches in diameter.

Place sausage patties on the unheated rack of a broiler pan. Broil 4 to 5 inches from the heat for 4 minutes. Turn and broil for 4 to 5 minutes more or till no longer pink. Pat sausage patties with paper towels. Arrange on a serving plate. Garnish with apple slices and fresh sage leaves, if desired. Makes 4 servings.

NUTRITION INFORMATION PER SERVING

73 calories, 0 g saturated fat, 0 g monounsaturated fat, 0 g polyunsaturated fat, 14 g protein, 3 g carbohydrate, 0 g dietary fiber, 36 mg cholesterol, 182 mg sodium, 148 mg potassium.

TURKEY CHILI

Nonstick spray coating
1   pound lean ground raw turkey
1   cup chopped celery
1   16 ounce can tomatoes, cut up
1   16 ounce can red kidney beans, drained
1   8 ounce can tomato sauce
1   6 ounce can vegetable juice cocktail
1   bay leaf
2   tablespoons minced onions
1 ½ teaspoon instant beef bouillon granules
1 ½ teaspoon ground cumin
¼   teaspoon garlic
¼   teaspoon crushed red pepper (option)
Toasted Pita chips

Spray a cold large skillet with nonstick coating. Add turkey and celery. Cook till turkey is no longer pink, stirring to break up pieces.

Stir in tomatoes; beans; tomato sauce, juice cocktail, bay leaf, onion, basil, bouillon granules, cumin, garlic, red pepper if desired, and ½ cup water. Bring to boiling, reduce heat. Simmer, uncovered, for 20 minutes, stirring occasionally. Discard bay leaf. Serve with toasted pita chips, if desired.

NUTRITION INFORMATION PER SERVING

380 calories, 4 g saturated fat, 5 g monounsaturated fat, 3 g polyunsaturated fat, 33 g protein, 3 g carbohydrate, 10 g dietary fiber, 71 mg cholesterol, 926 mg sodium, 1,272 mg potassium

CHAPTER 15 | EATING A BALANCED MEAL

TOASTED PITA CHIPS

4 pita bread crumbs
Split each pita horizontally in half. Cut each half into 6 wedges. Spread in a single layer on a baking sheet. Bake in a 350 degree oven about 10 minutes or till crisp. Serve warm. Serves 4.

NUTRITION INFORMATION PER SERVING
165 calories, 0 g saturated fat, 0 g monounsaturated fat, 0 g polyunsaturated fat, 6 g protein, 33 g carbohydrate, 1 g dietary fiber, 0 mg cholesterol, 339 mg sodium, 71 mg potassium.

SWEET AND SOUR TURKEY

Nonstick spray coating
4 turkey breast tenderloin steaks, cut ½ inch thick (about 1 pound)
½ of a 6 ounce can (1/3 cup) frozen pineapple juice concentrate, thawed
¼ cup water
¼ cup red wine vinegar
1 tablespoon soy sauce
¼ teaspoon garlic powder
¼ teaspoon ground ginger
2 tablespoons cold water
1 tablespoon cornstarch
1 11 ounce can mandarin orange sections drained
1 6 ounce package frozen pea pods
Tomato wedges (optional)

Spray a cold large skillet with nonstick coating. Preheat skillet over medium heat, then add turkey steaks. Cook over medium heat for 5 to 7 minutes or till turkey is light brown, turning steaks once.

Meanwhile, for sauce, in a small bowl stir together pineapple juice concentrate, water, vinegar, soy sauce, garlic powder, and ginger.

Add sauce to skillet. Bring to boiling; reduce heat. Simmer, covered, for 12 to 15 minutes or till turkey is no longer pink. Transfer turkey steaks to serving platter. Cover to keep warm.

In a custard cup stir together water and cornstarch. Stir mixture into sauce in the skillet. Cook and stir over medium heat till the mixture is thickened and bubbly.

Stir orange sections and frozen pea pods into mixture in the skillet. Cook and stir about 2 minutes or till heated through. Spoon oranges, pea pods, and sauce over turkey steaks. Garnish with tomato wedges, if desired. Makes 4 servings.

NUTRITION INFORMATION PER SERVING

226 calories, 0 g saturated fat, 0 g monounsaturated fat, 0 g polyunsaturated fat, 28 g protein, 27 g carbohydrate, 3 g dietary fiber, 71 mg cholesterol, 308 mg sodium, 512 mg potassium.

LIME-GLAZED TURKEY

¼ teaspoon finely shredded lime peel or lemon peel
2 tablespoons lime juice or lemon juice
1 tablespoon corn syrup
1 ¼ teaspoon dried tarragon, crushed
¼ teaspoon paprika
1/8 teaspoon salt
1/8 teaspoon garlic
Several dashes bottled hot pepper sauce
4 turkey breast tenderloin steaks, cut ½ inch thick

For glaze, in a small bowl combine lime or lemon juice, corn syrup, tarragon, paprika, salt, garlic powder, and hot pepper sauce. Mix well.

Rinse turkey and pat dry. Cook on an uncovered grill directly over medium coals for 6 minutes. Turn and brush with glaze. Continue cooking for 6 to 9 minutes more or till tender and no longer pink, brushing frequently with glaze during the last few minutes.

Or, to broil, place on the unheated rack of a broiler pan. Broil 4 to 5 inches from the heat for 5 minutes. Brush turkey with glaze. Turn and brush again with glaze. Continue broiling for 6 to 8 minutes more or till tender and no longer pink, brushing frequently with glaze during the last few minutes. Makes 4 servings.

NUTRITION INFORMATION PER SERVING
150 calories, 0 g saturated fat, 0 g monounsaturated fat, 0 g polyunsaturated fat, 26 g protein, 4 g carbohydrate, 0 g dietary fiber, 71 mg cholesterol, 124 mg sodium, 271 mg potassium.

CHERRY CHICKEN

2 whole medium chicken breasts (about 1 ½ pounds total), skinned, boned, and halved lengthwise, or 4 turkey breast tenderloin steaks, cut ½ inch thick
1 tablespoon lemon juice
1/3 cup cherry or seedless red raspberry preserves
1 tablespoon lemon juice
Dash ground allspice

Rinse chicken or turkey; pat dry. Place on the unheated rack of a broiler pan. Broil 4 to 5 inches from the heat for 6 minutes. Brush with some of the lemon juice. Turn poultry over. Brush, with remaining lemon juice. Broil 6 to 9 minutes or till tender and no longer pink.

For sauce, in a small saucepan cook and stir the preserves, lemon juice, and allspice over low heat till melted. Remove from heat. Pass sauce with chicken or turkey. Makes 4 servings.

NUTRITION INFORMATION PER SERVING

183 calories, 1 g saturated fat, 1 g monounsaturated fat, 1 g polyunsaturated fat, 20 g protein, 19 g carbohydrate, 0 g dietary fiber, 54 mg cholesterol, 52 mg sodium, 191 mg potassium.

VEGETABLE LASAGNA

6 lasagna noodles
2 slightly beaten egg whites
1 ½ cups low-fat cottage cheese, drained
1 10 ounce package frozen chopped broccoli or one 9-ounce package frozen French style green beans

Chapter 15 | Eating a Balanced Meal

4   green onions, sliced
¼   cup water
1   cup skim milk
4   teaspoons cornstarch
½   teaspoon dilled dill weed
    Dash pepper
1   cup shredded part-skim mozzarella cheese 4 ounces
    Nonstick spray coating
½   cup grated parmesan cheese

- Cook lasagna noodles according to package directions. Drain. Rinse with cold water. Drain again, set aside.
- Stir together egg whites, cottage cheese, and 1/8 teaspoon pepper. Set aside.
- Cook broccoli or green beans according to package directions. Drain, set aside.
- For sauce, in a medium saucepan cook green onions in water, covered, about 3 minutes or till tender.
- Combine skim milk, cornstarch, dill weed, and pepper.
- Add all at once to green onion mixture.
- Cook and stir till bubbly. Cook and stir for 1 minute more.
- Gradually add mozzarella cheese, stirring till melted.
- Stir in broccoli or green beans.
- Spray a 10x6x2 inch baking dish with nonstick coating. Place two of the noodles in the dish (if necessary, cut noodles to fit dish).
- Spread one third of the cottage cheese mixture over noodles.
- Top with on third of the sauce.
- Then, sprinkle with one-third of the parmesan cheese.
- Repeat layers 2 more times. Cover the dish with foil.
- Bake in a 350 degree oven for 30 minutes.
- Remove foil.
- Bake for 5 to 10 minutes more or till heated through.
- Let stand 10 minutes before serving.

Makes 6 servings.

Before you start to assemble the lasagna, measure the noodles against the dish. If the noodles are longer than the dish, use scissors to trim them to fit. Start with a layer of noodles in the bottom of the dish. Then, top with layers of the cottage cheese mixture, the sauce, and the parmesan cheese. Repeat these layers two more time.

NUTRITION INFORMATION PER SERVING

264 calories, 4 g saturated fat, 2 g monounsaturated fat, 0 g polyunsaturated fat, 23 g protein, 26 g carbohydrate, 2 g dietary fiber, 57 mg cholesterol, 497 mg sodium, 327 mg potassium.

Recipes from Better Homes and Garden Healthy Heart Cooking Ideas LOW-FAT FAVORITES

Note: Dr. Askar has been using these recipes since 1991

"I made a lot of friends over the years and I would always look at what they were eating. All of them were skinny. I would think that I would like to eat like that."
Suzanne Somers

Chapter Sixteen

How Stress Affects Weight Loss
By Brady Schuyler, DC

How Stress Affects Weight Loss
By Brady Schuyler, DC

Research has shown that stress has many adverse effects on the body. In this section we are going to discuss exactly how stress affects the body; and more importantly, how excess stress makes it more difficult to control weight.

What is Stress?

Stress can be defined as any physical, chemical, emotional, or psychological experience that forces your body to make a change. Stresses can be good or bad depending on how they force the body to change.

Some stresses, called eustress, are generally good for you. Physical exercise, mental challenges and gratifying emotions are all types of eustress that promote positive, healthy changes in the body.

Acute stress is another type of stress that we encounter, which may be the result of a short-term, serious, or potentially life threatening situation. This is typically known as the "stress response" or "fight or flight response". Our bodies are wired to respond immediately to certain situations, but it takes a huge amount of energy and resources to respond to this type of stress.

Chronic Stress is the type that we most often consider stress. These are the stresses of a job, the pressure of raising a family, financial concerns, unhealthy diets, and a sedentary lifestyle. This type of stress elicits the same response as the acute stresses, but is generally not as exhaustive. However, over time, chronic stress will eventually lead to burnout.

When a stress is perceived by your senses, your conscious or subconscious mind has to determine how it is going to respond to the stress. This is a very important thought process because it implies that our response to a given situation is a choice. What is a very critical situation to one person may be a mere inconvenience to another. That means that our response to a particular situation may determine what type of stress is perceived and how our body responds to it. So what exactly happens in our body when we experience stress?

The Role of Hormones In Stress

Our body's response to stress is controlled by our nervous system. A part of our nervous system, called the autonomic nervous system, sends a signal to our brain to alert us about a stressful situation. That part of the brain, called the hypothalamus, sends a signal via the hypothalamic-pituitary axis (HPA) to a small set of glands on the kidneys called the adrenal glands. These glands produce and release adrenaline and cortisol (and many other hormones) into the blood stream in response to that stress. These hormones travel throughout the body with one goal--to prepare the body to respond to the stressful encounter.

Is Your Stress Response Normal?

An acute stress response, or fight-or-flight response, is a completely normal and essential reaction that our body must go through to have the energy and resources readily available for a stressful encounter. It isn't until the acute stress response becomes stimulated over a prolonged period of time to chronic stressors that the long-term effects of the stress hormones start to take a toll on the body. Furthermore, these small little adrenal glands that secrete the hormones of adrenaline and cortisol (among other hormones) cannot keep up with the demands of the chronic stresses our body is exposed to which leads to burnout or "adrenal fatigue." This process was popularized in the 1950's by the work of Hans Selye and his concept of the General Adaptation Syndrome.

Just as important as understanding that exposure to chronic stress ultimately leads to adrenal fatigue, is what happens throughout the body when exposed to the stress hormones over prolonged periods. Again, this is a completely essential response to a short term acute stressor, but over longer periods, this same response leads to what Selye called the "Diseases of Adaptation." Our bodies are programmed to respond to the demands put on it and will always attempt to adapt to the conditions it is exposed to. However, under prolonged, non-life threatening chronic stresses, the body fails to adapt any longer and the essential, intelligent response becomes an illness or disease.

We are going to go over the various parts of the body in which the stress hormones have a direct effect. Again, this is the "fight or flight response" which is supposed to prepare your body for an extreme, potentially life threatening situation. For each organ or system that is covered, we will look at both the essential intelligent, short-term response to an acute stressor, as well as the prolonged, negative, disease-causing effects from the exposure to chronic stress. This is a very brief, simplified version explained by Dr. James L. Chestnut, B.Ed, MSc, DC, The Wellness Practice.

As previously discussed, when your senses perceive a

threat, or stressful situation, your brain signals for the release of stress hormones, including adrenaline and cortisol, into the bloodstream which has the following short-term and long-term effects:

Heart and Circulation:

- *Speeds up the heart rate and increases blood pressure to get the blood, which carries oxygen and other nutrients, to the parts of the body that use a lot of energy. It also stimulates the production of clotting factors in case you are wounded.*
- *Leads to chronic high blood pressure and atherosclerosis*

Liver:

- *Slows down the production of "good" cholesterol, and increase the amount of "bad" cholesterol. HDL cholesterol is a storage molecule and LDL is a more readily usable form. Cholesterol is used throughout the body for wound repair, hormone production, and mood regulation.*
- *Causes high cholesterol (the "bad" kind)*

Blood Glucose Levels:

- *Increased through a few different ways to provide quick energy throughout the body. Glycogen is broken down into glucose in the liver to increase levels. Insulin resistance is increased so glucose cannot be removed from the bloodstream.*
- *High levels of glucose stimulate the pancreas to produce more insulin. Eventually the pancreas cannot keep up and you develop type II diabetes.*

Immune System:

- *During an acute stress response, it is not necessary for your body to put a lot of energy into building a strong immune system. Cortisol decreases the rate at which immune cells are produced.*
- *Chronic Stress makes it more difficult to stay healthy and fight off infections.*

Emotional Centers:

- *Following an acute stress response, serotonin is released to calm your body down from the stressful encounter.*
- *Chronic stress makes your body continuously release serotonin until it cannot keep up with the demands. Over time, serotonin levels drop and you have difficulty recovering from the stressors. This leads to anxiety, difficulty sleeping, excess tension, and lowered sex drive.*

Increased Appetite:

- *Your appetite is stimulated to crave the building blocks of stress hormone, fats and sugar, to help your body keep up with the production of more hormones.*
- *Leads to overeating of less healthy foods which your body stores as fat.*

Looking at all of these changes that occur with the body under chronic stress, isn't it easy to see how we put on a few pounds in response? Chronic stress is not something our bodies were ever designed to deal with. The acute stress response, or *"fight or flight response,"* is an innate survival mechanism that helps you get through certain situations, but the chronic levels are something our bodies were never intended to handle.

Excess weight is a cumulative result of the chronic stress loads that our body shouldn't have to deal with. Excess weight is not something that our bodies would intelligently choose to have. The body storing excess weight is the result of the dysfunctional changes that occur as the result of chronic stress.

Stress's Devastating Effects

So now that we understand that the changes that occur in the body to an acute stress are intelligent and essential, chronic stress often has devastating effects that lead to illness and disease. Many times it is not that our bodies break down for no specific reason, it is that they cannot keep up with the demands that are required to function under these conditions.

A Past Metaphor to Understand Stress Better

Let's think about a struggling plant. How many of you have ever had a plant that started to wilt or droop? If you walk into a room and see one of your plants not looking very healthy, what is the first thing you are going to check? The first and most logical answer is the water, right? You check the water and the soil seems to be damp.

What else might you check? The sunlight? Is it getting too much sun or not enough sun? What if that is not the issue? What else might you look at? Add some plant food? Check to see if it is outgrowing the pot? Maybe the soil got contaminated with something?

The point is, when a plant is struggling and starting to show the effects of a stressed environment, we ask the right questions, *"What is this plant not getting that it needs?"* or *"What is this plant getting that it doesn't need?"*

Depriving, a plant of water, oxygen, sunlight, or nutrients is a stress to the plant. However, if you give the plant too much water, light, or nutrients, that could be a stress as well. If any of those conditions are maintained for a prolonged period, the plant will die. We are smart enough to understand the basic requirements of a plant, but we don't always ask the same question of ourselves when our bodies are showing signs of chronic stress.

Three Questions to Ask Yourself

1. *What are the basic requirements your body needs to survive and thrive?*
2. *What are you giving your body that it doesn't need?*
3. *What aren't you giving your body that it does need?*

To answer these questions we have to understand the different areas of our lives that have the potential to add to the chronic stress levels we are concerned about.

The Three Common Areas of Stress

These three areas can all contribute to chronic stress levels: physical, chemical, and psychological/emotional stresses. We are exposed to stress from each of these areas at all times but occasionally stress from one area may dominate our lives due to specific experiences and may cause excessive levels of stress on our systems. You may feel that one particular physical, chemical or psychological/emotional stress may always dominate your life and be the cause of your problems. However, it is most commonly combinations from all three areas at varying levels that create the chronic elevated levels in the body.

Similar to the stresses in the plant, as we look at each of these areas and how they relate to our lives there can be stresses of excess and stresses of deficiency. Let's go through and identify some of the different causes of physical, chemical and psychological/emotional stress.

Physical stresses that elicit the stress response can be a result of moving too much, moving not enough, or moving inefficiently. You can actually have stress from over-activity, but this tends to be an acute stress and the body's response and adaptation to the activity tends to be beneficial. More commonly, when joints and muscles are not moving the way they are supposed to, the stress response is stimulated. This could be due to bad posture, past injuries, muscular compensations or lack of overall use.

Chemical causes of stress, again, can be from not getting enough of what we need or getting too much of substances we don't need. How many of us get the recommend dose of 5-9 servings of fruits and vegetables per day? Are you eating the foods to supply all the other essential vitamins and minerals to keep up with the requirements of your body? How many things do you put into your body that it doesn't need?

How is the quality of the air you breathe on a daily basis? Are we getting fresh air or subjecting our bodies to the more prevalent, low-quality indoor air from our homes and work place. Are we using medications, both prescription and over-the-counter, to treat illness or symptoms of disease? All of these variables (and many more) are potential contributors to chemical strain on the body and stimulants of the stress response.

Probably the easiest to identify but the most difficult to do much about are the psychological/emotional stresses. These are typically what most people consider stress, when this should really be considered anxiety. We do not have to describe many of these in detail because anyone can probably come up with their own more complete, all-inclusive list than I could.

Rarely is anxiety a beneficial emotion but remember stresses are not only those of excess but also of lack. Some essential positive psychological/emotional stresses are commonly missing such as: mental challenge or stimulation, feelings of love and being loved, appreciation, and the ability to relax and feel pleasure.

Ask yourself, what is right for me?

How can I examine these areas of my life and assess the levels of stress that I am getting from each area? Are you thinking to yourself, "Well, I eat really well and I exercise. So I am ok in the physical and chemical areas of my life. It's just the psychological/emotional stress."

Rarely is anyone so extremely balanced in one or two of these areas, while so overloaded in the other that it creates the chronic levels associated with illness or disease. That's not to say that this cannot occur, because it would give a rational explanation to the guy who looks healthy and has a daily exercise regimen, yet falls over with a sudden fatal heart attack.

Do we know what this person's emotional stress levels are? Many of us have heard stories of people, who seem apparently healthy, yet a chronic illness or disease develops.

Even though a person may be extremely physically active and may even eat very well, could they have extremely high levels of anxiety? Could they have been dealing with so much anxiety and emotional stress that it was enough to drive the stress response and the body to the point of fatigue or dysfunction of heart or circulatory system as discussed previously?

Ask, how does this apply to me?

The real question is, "Are you happy with where you are or do you want to change?" Is what you are telling yourself mentally consistent with what you are doing physically, chemically and emotionally? You learned that stress from anyone of those three areas can contribute to overall stress levels in the body, so even if you can't make changes in one area that you know is very difficult for you, you can work on the other 2 areas to lower the overall cumulative level. If emotional stress is something you cannot seem to get away from in this stage of your life then--as much as you can--improve the physical and chemical levels of stress that you are able to control and impact.

How much is enough?
How much should I strive to improve?

That is all relative. If you take someone who is 75 pounds overweight and has been sedentary and asked them to walk 1 mile 3 times a week, it could be nearly impossible. If you take a highly trained athlete who works out 6 days week doing a variety of workouts and tell them they can only walk 1 mile 3 times a week, they will bounce off the wall.

A simple philosophy is to imagine a healthy person.

- *How do they live? How do they eat?*
- *What kind of activities do they do?*
- *What are their hobbies?*
- *Do you want to be that person?*
- *Are your actions consistent with those thoughts?*

You now know that the acute stress response is an intelligent normal response your body goes through to handle certain situations.

You also understand how high levels of chronic stress stimulate this same response, which can fatigue systems in your body and can negatively affect your health.

You can identify physical, chemical, and psychological/emotional contributors in your life--those of too much of what you don't need and those of not enough of what you need.

Ultimately, if you are not happy with your current situation, look for areas to improve. Health and ideal weight is not black and white. You can always strive toward better health and your ideal weight by identifying the different areas of stress in your life and finding ways to improve them.

CHAPTER SEVENTEEN

Brain Neurotransmitters and Hormones
By Steven R. Troeger, D.C.
and Deborah L. Troeger, M.A.

Brain Neurotransmitters and Hormones
Steven R. Troeger, D.C. and
Deborah L. Troeger, M.A.

What are Neurotransmitters?

Most of us have never heard of neurotransmitters, or are, at least, not very familiar with what they really are and do. You are probably familiar with hormones and what they do, but maybe not the ones we'll talk about here. I'm not talking about just the sex hormones, but the ones that drive our metabolism in particular.

In this chapter we would like to give you an understanding of how these brain controlling chemicals affect you and, most importantly, how you can affect them and how you feel. Despite what we may think, we really are in control of our bodies. Every day you make decisions as to what your body needs and wants. Unfortunately, many of those decisions will not help your health or make you feel good in the long run. By reading this chapter, you're giving yourself the opportunity to take control and give yourself the best chance at good body composition and health.

Let's start with a bit of an analogy to help you understand just how our hormones and neurotransmitters work and how we can affect them with not only the food we eat, but the way we put that food together during our day. Most of us have driven a car or at least are pretty familiar with how they work. We all know that to run they must have fuel--in the car's case, gasoline.

We also know that we have a choice of fuels to pick

Chapter 18 | High Tech Solution To Weight Loss

from at the pump. Our Chevy Impala's info book says we should use 85 octane gasoline. We bought this car in the Mile High city of Denver where the air is thinner than it is at sea level.

So our mechanic put in new jets to deliver more fuel to the engine. He set the engine to run on a perfect mix of gasoline and air to give us the highest level of performance for where we lived. Then, later on, we moved to a new place that was on sea level. We didn't really think about the car. It was stressful enough just moving, adjusting to a new job, house and all. But then, I began to notice that the gas mileage was falling a bit--then more and more. I mistakenly thought that here at sea level, with more air, I should get better gas mileage.

First, I figured that I just needed to use a richer fuel with a higher octane rating. So I switched to premium. That didn't help the gas mileage, and I soon noticed that the tail pipe on my car was getting very black. Deciding to consult a professional, I went to visit my new mechanic. He explained to me that the proper mix of fuel and air was necessary to make the car run well. I was running "rich" with too much gas and not enough air and that the extra fuel that was not burning completely was showing up on my tailpipe as that black stuff.

Not only that, but it was doing the same thing inside my engine to the spark plugs. As a result, they were also very inefficient at burning fuel. He also explained that the opposite can be true, that if we run "lean"--not enough fuel for the amount of air--that the engine can seem to perform better for a while but in fact the engine runs hotter and can burn my cylinder heads. Big problem and expensive repairs!

So, the "cure" for my engine was to use the recommended octane of fuel for my engine and to have the jets replaced with ones that would allow the proper air fuel mix. Since doing that, my car runs better, idles better, gets good gas mileage and just seems to be happier. It seems to run better when I wash it as well and replace the air cleaner and fuel filter periodically.

Now that we are all up on how to take care of our cars, what does that have to do with brain neurotransmitters and hormones? Our bodies work much the same way. We have to take care of them in the correct combinations for them to be happy and run efficiently.

What do Hormones Have to Do With It?

First, some information on exactly which chemicals we are talking about. Let's start with the hormones--insulin, thyroid, testosterone, estrogen, growth hormone and glucagon. Insulin is probably the first hormone we think of when we talk about body composition and our health. Most of us know that insulin is the hormone related to blood sugar and diabetes, but how does it work and what affects it? Insulin helps our body by pushing glycogen and blood sugar into our muscle cells so that we have a supply of energy to fuel our muscle activity.

When we eat, our blood sugar rises and we produce insulin in the pancreas to keep the blood sugar at a safe level. We do that by pushing and storing the glycogen into the muscle. However, if we eat more carbohydrate than we need, we produce more glycogen than we can store in the muscle.

Then we push the sugar to the liver and we store it as fat. Insulin is both lipogenic, (makes fat), and antilipolytic, (stops the breakdown of fat). Insulin also has many other negative effects on our bodies when it is present in greater quantities than we should have. As the saying goes, can't live with too much of it and can't live without it. It's all about balance!

Influences On Our Hormones

When we are under stress, especially for extended periods of time, we produce a stress hormone called cortisol, which also causes an increase in the production of insulin. Not only is that bad news for us, but cortisol also causes a decrease in the production of DHEA, which is helpful in making muscle.

We now know that the abdominal fat cells have a higher level of cortisol response than other fat cells and as a result, especially with long term stress, we get more fat deposition in our abdominal areas. So, to avoid the decreased muscle, decreased energy burn, increased fat storage (most markedly around our bellies), insulin must be controlled as tightly as possible.

Most of us have heard of thyroid hormone. The thyroid is a small gland in our neck that is responsible for producing a hormone that works as our body's thermostat. It helps keep us warm and maintain our body temperature.

It does this by telling us how much energy to burn to keep us at a healthy 98.6 degrees no matter what situation we are in. Thyroxine increases our BMR (Basal Metabolic Rate) and increases up to 30% with exercise, helping us to burn those stored calories.

Sometimes we develop problems and our thyroid doesn't do its job. Most commonly, it becomes sluggish and we begin to see symptoms like low energy, fatigue, constipation, depression, lethargy, increased cholesterol, dry skin and hair, decreased fat burning and weight gain. Physicians often test blood for thyroid problems but unfortunately, these lab tests seem to be very unreliable unless the thyroid is severely deficient in function.

Estrogen is obviously produced in greater quantities in women, but men produce it as well. There are three forms of estrogen but we will talk briefly about only one-- 17 beta estradiol, the most active form. Estrogen increases fat breakdown. It also increases our BMR and elevates our mood and libido. Estrogen increases with exercise.

As women near menopause and they naturally decrease their production of estrogen, they are often placed on hormone replacement therapy to simulate the missing estrogen and as a result seem to gain weight as body fat. We believe that this is due to the often severe imbalance between estrogen and progesterone. It seems that hormone replacement therapy (and oral contraceptives) often stimulate the appetite and cause weight /fat gain.

We also see increased fat levels when we take in estrogen mimickers that may be found in plastics and many chemicals. These estrogen mimickers and xenoestrogens can be very deleterious to our health in general and are very disruptive to cellular health. We believe that this is one of the reasons for the increasing weight problems seen in our young children today. It has become very difficult to control the intake of these chemicals and as a result of this increase in ingested chemicals, we suffer many symptoms of hormone imbalance.

Testosterone is the male hormone, but as with estrogen, we all make some. Testosterone maintains our muscle mass, helps us build muscle and builds muscle strength. This increases our BMR and allows us to consume more calories and continue to burn them more efficiently. Testosterone decreases our body fat, increases our self confidence and increases our libido and intensity of orgasms. It decreases for females near menopause and typically begins to decline in men in their forties. Like estrogen, you can increase testosterone levels with exercise.

Growth hormone does just what it says it will do. It stimulates growth and stimulates protein synthesis. It decreases the use of glucose for energy and increases the utilization of fat for energy. This would have the obvious effect of reducing your body fat; and in so doing, it increases the amount of time that you can exercise by keeping your blood sugar levels more balanced and normal.

Release of growth hormone from the pituitary gland is stimulated by aerobic exercise and is increased by upping your time and intensity of exercise. The bad news is that the older we get the less growth hormone we produce, but that doesn't mean you can't continue to do some good, regular aerobic exercise, right?

Finally, let's spend a bit of time on a hormone most people are not familiar with--glucagon. After our short discussion, you will probably be quite fond of glucagon and what it does. We often think of glucagon as the balancer of insulin. Glucagon is also a pancreatic-produced hormone just like insulin. Its job is to raise the blood sugar level for our utilization by returning fat to the liver and converting it to glucose.

It releases fat for energy, whereas insulin stores fat by conversion in the liver. Glucagon is released after about 30 minutes of exercise when the muscle stores of glycogen begin to go down and our blood sugar begins to fall a bit. Glucagon is a major key to why Atkins type diets are effective.

What About Serotonin and Your Adrenal Glands?

For most of us these names may not be so familiar and how they actually affect us may be even less well known. Brain neurotransmitters basically direct how we feel and, as a result, how we respond to situations like stress, sadness, joy and anger. Often our appetites are directly affected by the way that we respond to these situations. Unfortunately, most of these responses are not exactly good for us.

Serotonin is a very powerful endorphin and can have affects that are crucial in our ability to control our weight. Low levels of serotonin can cause depression, lethargy and an increased desire for carbohydrates. It seems that low levels of serotonin tell our body's systems that we are in a time of famine and that we need to eat and store more calories. We think we're starving and we have an increased appetite.

High stress and/or prolonged stress causes an increase in cortisol as we mentioned earlier, which also causes a decrease in serotonin. This may trigger an increased intake of refined carbohydrates, or ice cream....what's your favorite?

Not getting enough protein in our diet or not having it balanced properly also seems to cause a decrease in serotonin. Proper balance of protein and carbohydrate will help balance serotonin and endorphin production. You can also increase your levels up to 5 times the resting levels by doing some good aerobic exercise for over 30 minutes at a moderate or above moderate intensity level.

If you exercise regularly, over time the endorphins stay in your system longer and you develop an increased sensitivity as well.

The adrenal glands are located on top of our kidneys and produce several very important and potent chemicals including cortisol, epinephrine and norepinephrine. As we know, cortisol is a stress hormone and can wreak havoc on our systems when it stays around for a long time. Epinephrine stimulates the breakdown of glycogen in active muscle tissues and the liver to burn it as fuel. It stimulates the breakdown and conversion of fat to glucose and is released proportionally to the amount and intensity of exercise.

Can You Control Your Weight With Neurotransmitters?

As you might have gathered during this rapid race through our hormones and some of the neurotransmitters, this is a very complicated system and might seem a bit overwhelming for us to apply to weight management. So what does it all mean? How do we use the knowledge to our advantage? Can we really control our weight using the concept of these chemicals beyond just eat less than you burn? Many people have said that a calorie is a calorie. We don't believe that for a minute. A calorie from a refined sugar will not do the same things in your body as a calorie from chicken. As we have said several times through the chapter, it's all about balance. We need a balance between insulin and glucagon and each of the other opposing hormones and neurotransmitters.

As in our car engine analogy, we must balance our air/gas mixture to have our engine run smoothly and efficiently. When we eat too many refined carbohydrates, we over stimulate the fat storage hormones. When we are stressed, especially for long periods of time, we stimulate the fat storage hormones. If our thyroid is low functioning but healthy, we stimulate fat storage. If our sex hormones are out of balance, we stimulate fat storage. If we are overstressed causing depression and lethargy, we stimulate fat storage.

If we want to have increased energy, increased fat burn, increased libido, increased muscle mass and increased feelings of wellbeing, we have to decrease the refined carbohydrate calories, increase the amount of good quality protein, maintain balance in each meal every day--including the eating of good omega 3 fats and the reduction of the omega 6 (vegetable oil) and trans fats. When we need to burn extra fat and reduce our body fat we use these chemicals to our advantage by changing the air/fuel mix for a period of time and then returning to the balance point when we get to our healthy weight.

Many have tried to use high protein type diets to stimulate fat burning, but find it impossible to maintain. This is due to our concept of balance being pushed way over the edge. Not enough of those endorphins are being produced to make us feel good and too many are produced that make us feel hyperactive and nervous. Some people are too stressed or depressed or too caught up in their life patterns to want to exercise and they don't change their diet to allow the production of stimulatory hormones.

These folks just seem to put on weight constantly without even trying. Many will tell you that they don't even eat very much and they probably don't--they are eating all the wrong foods and stimulating all the wrong hormones and neurotransmitters. Their bodies are just following the chemical instructions they are giving.

What Can You Expect When Supplementing With Amino Acids?

Unlike some medications used to alter and enhance mood--which can take months to notice any positive change--amino acids effects can be noticed sometimes within hours or just a few days. Some people have described the effect as if a dark cloud had been lifted. They had not changed anything else in their lives, but after taking the amino acids their world seemed brighter and hopeful. For a lot of people making dietary changes affects and improves energy level and mood.

Some people claim they just do not have the "willpower" to eliminate the refined carbohydrates in their diets. We have found that if you are significantly depleted in some of these amino acids, your body is going to crave certain foods to artificially create the chemical reactions it needs to function that normally it would get if the amino acids were present. So, it may not be that you are lacking willpower, it may just mean that your body is craving certain foods for a reason and by adding the appropriate amino acids you can help balance your body chemistry and eliminate the cravings.

It takes significant energy--emotional, mental and physical--to make changes. Experts say that the first several minutes of take off on the space shuttle requires more fuel than the entire rest of the trip. The same is true in changes we make in our lives. The first 28 days takes energy to plan, prepare, and follow the plan. Some people that we have worked with are so easily overwhelmed that just the thought of taking some nutritional snacks to work seems like way too much to think about, let alone add 20-30 min of exercise to the mix.

It may be a relief to know that maybe it isn't that you are too lazy or have no willpower. You could be lacking the amino acid that, when low, creates side effects that are overwhelming. Here is what Kim, one of our patients, had to say about her experience with amino acids, " Dr. Troeger first suggested I take L-tyrosine about a year ago when it felt like regardless of the amount of sleep I got I was exhausted. I now take 3 tablets in the morning right after breakfast and now I feel great all day. I have the energy to get through the day without any of the jittery side effects associated with other options like caffeine."

The good news is that if you do find yourself scoring high on the questionnaire that we supply later in this chapter, the use of amino acid supplements may help prime your body to produce more. (You might want to seek out a physician who works with amino acids to help monitor and suggest doses).

Most people find that they do not need to continue taking them forever to achieve optimum results--unlike antidepressants and other medications. Once you get the balance back, combined with proper diet and exercise, you can maintain optimum mood, body function, energy levels and weight!

Unfortunately, our body is unlike our car in the earlier analogy and it cannot be replaced. If you abuse your car or don't maintain it properly, you can just go get a new one. You might get a new one just because you feel like it! You can't do that with your body!

You might think that it would be easier to just get liposuction or gastric bypass surgery. That may work for a while, but if you continue with the same bad habits and do not solve what is causing the cravings, at some point your body will adjust and find a way to get those calories in and the pounds will come right back on.

Many people who have had the lap band or gastric bypass end up replacing "donuts" for other refined, often liquid, carbohydrates, and within 5 years they are back where they started. It is important to pay attention to the red warning lights on the dashboard of your car. By the time that light comes, on there has been a problem under the hood for some time.

The same is true for your body. By the time you are feeling sluggish, run down, depressed, unmotivated, unable to focus, etc.… there has been a problem in your body for a long time. If you just continue to ignore the symptoms and make excuses, the problem will not go away. *It runs in my family. I'm just not motivated. I'm getting old. If only …* Excuses will only turn into larger problems like diabetes, heart disease, metabolic syndrome, cancer…

It's Too Bad We Don't have Warning Lights

What would happen if your check-engine light goes unchecked for months or maybe even years. At some point the engine would probably just blow up and quit running. You could be like Homer Simpson and just put some duct tape over the light and assume that because you can't see it, it's okay.

A lot of people do that. They take medication, have liposuction, eat more comfort food, drink alcohol, sleep more. Whatever the band aid, the effect is the same. At some point your body will "blow up" and unfortunately there is no "cash for clunkers" program available for us!

Quick Tips For Neurotransmitters in Weight Management.

Tip #1 Find creative ways to deal with stress. Practice the techniques found in Chapter 10 and 16 and use your Behavioral Repatterning Device.

Tip #2 Cut back on refined carbohydrates and artificial sweeteners. Studies show that people who use artificial sweeteners actually gain more weight and eat more than those who don't.

Tip #3 Avoid caffeine. Caffeine also stimulates insulin production and even though there may be no calories in the caffeinated drinks, they actually tell your body to store more fat. You may feel like you need an extra pick-me-up in the afternoon and reaching for a "high octane" caffeinated drink may seem like a good idea at the time. However, it may actually cause a huge crash later in the day requiring more stimulation and increasing fat storage.

Tip #4 Stick to the whole grains. Eat good quality protein to stimulate dopamine and norepinephrine to increase your energy, alertness and ability to focus.

Tip #5 Exercise regularly to stimulate energy, alertness, focus, fat burn, muscle increase and increasing those feel good endorphins. You may have noticed the many references to 20-30 minutes of aerobic exercise throughout the chapter.

Tip #6 Get checked. Balance between testosterone, estrogen and progesterone is important and changes through our lives and life stresses.

Tip #7 Steroids, antidepressants, diabetic medications, NSAID's and other drugs can cause weight gain and fluid retention.

Tip #8 Finally, we have found that in many of our patients, the balance of brain neurotransmitters that are affected by diet and particularly protein intake and digestion, need to be supplemented with amino acids to help the body return to proper brain chemical balance. We have included a copy of Julia Ross's Amino Acid Questionnaire to help you understand how these key neurotransmitters affect you and may be balanced to increase your ability to manage your weight effectively

Chapter 17 | Understanding the Neurotransmitters and Hormones that Affect Weight Control

Which Carb-Addicted Brain Type Are You?
IDENTIFY AND ELIMINATE FALSE APPETITES, FALSE WEIGHT AND FALSE MOODS

TYPE 1 Low in SEROTONIN *(our natural antidepressant)*
- ❒ negativity, depression
- ❒ worry, anxiety
- ❒ low self-esteem
- ❒ repetitious, obsessive thoughts or behaviors
- ❒ hyperactivity
- ❒ fear of heights, water, snakes, performance, etc.
- ❒ benefits from anti-depressant drugs
- ❒ panic attacks
- ❒ winter blues (SAD)
- ❒ suicidal thoughts
- ❒ fibromyalgia, TMJ, migraines
- ❒ irritability, rage
- ❒ night-owl, insomnia, disturbed sleep, hard to get to sleep
- ❒ dislike hot weather
- ❒ afternoon or evening cravings for sweets, starches, alcohol, or cannabis

Solution: 5-HTP 50 mg or l-tryptophan 500 mg (1-3) mid-afternoon & evening.

TYPE 2 Low in CATECHOLEMINE *(our natural stimulant)*
- ❒ cravings for sweets, chocolate, caffeine, or other stimulants for a lift
- ❒ depressed, bored, apathetic
- ❒ lack of energy, drive
- ❒ lack of focus, concentration, A.D.D.

Solution: L-Tyrosine 500 mg (1-3) on arising and mid-morning (and mid-afternoon if no insomnia)

TYPE 3 Low in GABA *(our natural tranquilizer)*
- ❒ cravings for sweets, starches, alcohol or tranquilizers when stressed
- ❒ over-stressed, burned out, overwhelmed
- ❒ unable to relax, loosen up, meditate, pray, slow down, sleep
- ❒ feel stiff and tense

Solution: GABA 100-500 mg as needed

TYPE 4 Low in ENDORPHIN *(our natural pain killer)*
- ❏ crave comforting or numbing "treats," i.e., sweets, starches, chocolate, bread, cheese
- ❏ sensitive to emotional pain or have had chronic physical pain
- ❏ cry or "tear up" easily, sad too often
- ❏ "Love" certain foods, drugs, or alcohol

Solution: Dl-Phenylalanine (DLPA) 500 mg (2-4) on arising, mid-morning, and mid-afternoon (or dphenylalanine if anxious (1-2) 500 mg, 2-3x/day). Free-form amino blend 700 mg before meals.

TYPE 5 Low in BLOOD SUGAR *(adequate brain glucose stabilizes mood & appetite)*
- ❏ cravings for sweets, starches, and/or alcohol (especially if a meal has been missed or delayed)
- ❏ irritable, shaky, stressed, headachey, if it's been too long between meals

Solution: L-glutamine 500 mg (2-3) on arising, between meals and at bedtime, or open capsule in mouth
for instant relief. Chromium 200 mcg (2) with each meal.

ESSENTIAL NUTRITIONAL SUPPORT FOR ALL TYPES

Multivitamin and Mineral (2-6/day); Vitamin C Ascorbate 2000 mg/day; Cod Liver Oil

Foods: a minimum of 3 meals/day, each containing 20-30 gm protein (e.g., a chicken breast, 3 eggs, 1 cup cottage cheese). no less than 4 cups low-carb vegetables/day, plus only healthy fats (butter, ghee, coconut or olive oil) and high-carb foods (fruit, beans, potatoes) as needed. Avoid sweetened and flour-based foods, allergy foods & caffeine.

For more information: DietCure.com, RecoverySystemsClinic.com (415-383-3611)

© 2008 Julia Ross, M.A., author of The Diet Cure and The Mood Cure. Permission to copy with acknowledgement

USING AMINO ACIDS: PRECAUTIONS

If you have: overactive thyroid (Grave's disease),
PKU (phenylketonuria) or Melanoma;
Do NOT take: L-tyrosine, DL-phenylalanine,
or L-phenylalanine[1]

Please consult a knowledgeable practitioner before taking any amino acids if any of the following statements apply to you:

❐ You react to supplements, foods or medications with unusual or uncomfortable symptoms

❐ You have serious physical illness, particularly cancer

❐ You have severe liver or kidney problems

❐ You have an ulcer (amino acids are slightly acidic)

❐ You are pregnant or nursing

❐ You have schizophrenia or other mental illness

❐ You are taking any medications for mood problems, particularly MAO inhibitors or more than one SSRI. You react to supplements, foods or medications with unusual or uncomfortable symptoms

Consult an expert before taking: If you have:	Melatonin	L-tyrosine or L-phenylalanine	GABA	5-HTP	DLPA	L-glutamine[1]
elevated cortisol (severe 2:-4:AM insomnia)				X		
asthma[2]	X			X		
high blood pressure		X			X	
low blood pressure			X			
tendency to get migraine headaches		X			X	
manic-depressive (bipolar) tendencies[3]	X				X	X

Even if your doctor agrees that you can try amino acids (or any other nutrients), if you experience discomfort of any kind after taking them, stop taking them immediately.

© Julia Ross, author of The Mood Cure (Penguin 2004) & The Diet Cure (Penguin 2000)

---

1) *In rare cases, glutamine might raise blood sugar in diabetics*
2) *Nocturnal asthma seems to be the primary problem. Tryptophan may also cause problems for asthmatics.*
3) *SAM-E, St. John's Wort, bright therapeutic lamps, chromium, and too much fish or flax oil may also trigger mania.*

CHAPTER EIGHTEEN

HIGH-TECH SOLUTIONS FOR HIGH-TECH STRESS
Patrick K. Porter, Ph.D.

High-Tech Solutions for High-Tech Stress
By Patrick K. Porter, Ph.D.

In the middle of a scorching summer heat wave, I attended a convention in Las Vegas, Nevada. It was only a few months after the opening of our new enterprise in Phoenix, and I really couldn't afford to be there. My curiosity got the better of me, however, when I discovered that new mind technology would be introduced at that event.

I was rushing to my next workshop when a female voice called out to me. I glanced at the woman who smiled at me as she stood in front of her booth. I waved and smiled at her. "I don't have time," I said. "I'm late for my next workshop."

Then a strange electronic device perched on the table behind her caught my eye. I touched the machine. "What's this?"

The woman stroked the device as if it were her beloved pet. "This is the Sensory Input Learning System. We call it SILS for short," she said. "I'm Linnea Reid." She shook my hand then signaled to a middle-aged man sitting beside the machine. "This is my partner, Larry Gillen," she added.

"Would you like to go for a ride?" Linnea asked.

One of my early loves was electronics, so I couldn't resist giving it a try. "Sure," I replied.

Linnea told me to lie back in a reclining chair. She tucked a blanket around me and handed me a set of earphones and a pair of sunglasses equipped with small LED lights. "I'll let you go about ten minutes," she said. "Just close your eyes and have a great trip."

Not knowing what to expect, I settled into the chair and closed my eyes. Within moments my senses were awakened by the rhythm of flashing lights and tones. An immediate feeling of relaxation and well-being washed over me. Now this was something I could get into.

By the time the session ended, I was blown away. I had never before felt so relaxed. I didn't want to move. "Come on," Linnea said as she shook me, "the group is about to take a break. You need to get up."

"That was the most amazing ten minutes of my life," I said.

"Ten minutes? That was more like forty-five minutes. You seemed to be having such a good time, I decided to let you keep going."

"Wow! It seemed to go that fast," I said, snapping my fingers. "I've got to have one of these machines. How do I buy one?"

"Well, you're in luck, I happen to sell these things… and the show special is only ten-thousand dollars."

My heart sank. I was a new business owner. She might as well have said ten million dollars. Yet I had never let money stand in my way before. I simply had to own one of these amazing devices. The wheels in my mind began to turn.

As fate would have it, Linnea and Larry relocated to Mesa, Arizona, and opened their business, Light & Sound Research, a short distance from my clinic. I attended several of their demonstrations and we soon formed a friendship.

One night, we sat in a diner discussing all the possibilities the SILS system offered. "I've got an idea," I said, "what if I sponsor your demonstrations at my clinic and, between events, you can leave the machine with me so I can research the benefits with my clients?"

"I have to admit, I'm pretty tired of hustling around to different locations," Larry said to Linnea. "Sounds like a great idea to me."

"I agree," she said. "Getting some feedback from real clients would be invaluable."

In that instant I had accomplished a goal without it costing me a dime. By setting no limitations on how I would possess the machine, I had visualized and realized my goal.

That was 1987. Since then almost every one of my clients, along with the clients who attended programs in my franchise system, experienced this life changing technology. To say the results were astounding would be an understatement.

How is technology changing the way we use our brain?

Light and sound technology, also known as visual/auditory entrainment, is introduced to the brain through the ears and optic nerve using computerized technology emitted through headphones and specially designed glasses equipped with light-emitting diodes (LEDs). The lights flash at predetermined frequencies and are coupled with binaural beats, which are heard at a low level through the headphones. The visual/auditory entrainment is typically synchronized, but can be varied depending on the desired effect.

The flickering light patterns and binaural beats reach the brain by way of the optic nerve and inner ear respectively. Within minutes the brain begins to match the frequencies of the light pulses and sound beats. The method by which this entrainment occurs is known as frequency following response. Unlike biofeedback, where the user attempts to consciously change brainwave activity, light and sound induced entrainment influences the brain without any conscious effort.

The frequency following response simulates the relaxed brainwave frequencies know as alpha and theta. This is the state in which the individual relaxes and the mind develops focus. Listeners experience a reduction in inner chatter and improved concentration. Because frequency following response is a learned response, the effect is cumulative. After a few weeks of regular use, users gain a sense of balance and inner calm. Most people report feeling serene, focused, and alert even when faced with high-pressure situations. Furthermore, most users report experiencing enhanced creativity and feeling more rested with less sleep. When we use this brainwave entrainment for changing habits, we call it behavioral repatterning.

While light and sound technology can be beneficial to most people, it is not for everyone. Persons with epilepsy, any type of seizure disorder, or any visual photosensitivity are advised against using a light and sound device. People who have a pacemaker, suffer from a heart disorder, have a history of serious head trauma, or are taking stimulants, tranquilizers, or psychotropic medications, including alcohol or drugs, should consult their physician before use. Anyone experiencing dizziness, migraine, or severe anxiety after using light and sound should discontinue using the device and consult a physician.

How do tones create relaxation?

In 1839, an associate professor at the University of Berlin, H. W. Dove, discovered what he termed binaural beats. His early research showed that putting a given frequency in one ear and a different tone in the other causes a person to hear a third tone, which is the difference in frequency of the two tones.

He found that the human ability to hear binaural beats appeared to be the result of evolutionary adaptation and that our brains detect and follow binaural beats because of the structure of the brain itself.

Until a 1973 article by Gerald Oster, however, binaural beats were considered no more than a scientific curiosity. Oster's paper was groundbreaking not so much in presenting new laboratory findings, but rather in bringing fresh insight to the topic by identifying and connecting a variety of relevant research performed after Dove's discovery.

Oster is credited with uncovering just what effect binaural beats could have on the mind and body. He viewed binaural beats as a tool for cognitive and neurological research. Moreover, he identified the auditory system's propensity for selective attention (sometimes referred to as the cocktail party effect), which is our ability to tune out distractions and focus on a single activity.

Oster also found that Parkinson's sufferers and those with auditory impairments generally could not hear binaural beats. Thus, he concluded that binaural beats could be used for diagnosing certain disorders. He also discovered gender differences in the perception of beats and felt that how a woman perceived the tones could be used to gauge fluctuations of estrogen (the latter assertion rising from a study he replicated that corroborated findings of gender differences in the perception of beats).

Oster's publication of "Auditory Beats in the Brain," along with his assertion that binaural beats could be created even when one of the frequencies is below the human volume threshold (which supported his hypothesis that binaural beats involved different neural pathways from those involved in our direct conscious perception), launched a wave of new research into frequency following response.

How Binaural Beats Work

1. *The binaural beat is generated from two separate tones of a slightly different pitch*
2. *One tone is presented to the left ear and the other to the right ear*
3. *Your brain combines the two tones to make a single new tone*
4. *The single tone pulses to match relaxed brainwave frequencies*
5. *Your brain follows the pattern and creates the relaxed state*

How does light create relaxation?

Almost since the time humans discovered fire, it's been observed that flickering light can cause alterations in consciousness and even inexplicable visual hallucinations. Throughout history, stories abound of tribal elders, healers, and shamans using this knowledge to enhance their practices.

Early scientists, also captivated by this phenomenon, explored its practical applications. Around 200 AD, Ptolemy experimented with a spinning spoked wheel placed between an observer and the sun. The flickering of the sunlight through the spokes of the spinning wheel caused patterns and colors to appear before the eyes of the observer. Many of these observers described a feeling of euphoria after exposure to the light patterns.

Joseph Plateau, a Belgian scientist, used the flickering of light through a strobe wheel to study the diagnostic significance of the flicker fusion phenomenon.

As he caused the light flickers to come faster and faster, he found that at a certain point the flickers seemed to "fuse" into a steady, unflickering light pattern. In 1829, Plateau dubbed this phenomenon persistence of vision.

He noted that healthy people were able to see separate flashes of light at much higher flicker speeds than were sick people. Today Plateau is recognized as the first animator. Modern filmmakers still rely on persistence of vision to trick our brains into believing that what we are viewing is actually moving and not just a series of still images.

At the turn of the century, French physician Pierre Janet noticed that when patients at the Salpetriere Hospital in Paris were exposed to flickering lights, they experienced reductions in hysteria and increases in relaxation.

By 1990, scientists were able to measure the effect of

light on serotonin and endorphin levels. In one such study, eleven patients had peridural (the outermost of the three membranes covering the brain and spinal cord) and blood analysis performed before and after participation in relaxation sessions using flash emitting goggles.

An average increase of beta-endorphin levels of twenty-five percent and serotonin levels of twenty-one percent were registered. The beta-endorphin levels are comparable to those obtained by cranial electrical stimulation (CES). The researchers concluded that photic stimulation has great potential for decreasing depression-related symptoms.

Four Brainwave Frequencies

Brainwave Frequency	Name
13–40 Hz	Beta waves (Reactionary Mind)

Active thought and concentration; associated with busyness and anxious thinking

7–13 Hz	Alpha waves (Intuitive Mind)

Relaxation (while awake), daydreaming; associated with creativity

4–7 Hz	Theta waves (Inventive Mind)

The place between asleep and awake; associated with deep meditation and sleep learning

< 4 Hz	Delta waves (Rejuvenating Mind)

Deep dreamless sleep

Chapter 18 | High Tech Solution To Weight Loss

Why use light and sound together?

While research has proven that both light (flickering) and sound (binaural beats) can produce relaxed states, at Light & Sound Research we found that combining the two could move the body into a more profound level of relaxation; it is the highly kinesthetic state of tranquility that is optimum for healing and accelerated learning.

When I met Linnea and Larry, it was at the dawn of the computer revolution. Microchip technology was in its infancy, and computer engineers were a rare commodity. Nevertheless, Larry and Linnea found an engineer who could program a computer chip to do the work that the therapist previously had to do. With the help of thousands of documented sessions using a mind mirror (EEG machine), they discovered which programs worked to optimize the frequency following response and bring about optimum states of relaxation and learning. They then designed the first portable relaxation system and called it the MC2.

In the next two decades, the franchise company I founded used this light and sound technology combined with behavioral repatterning to help hundreds of thousands of people facilitate life changes such as losing weight, kicking a smoking habit, or conquering an alcohol or drug addiction. Others used it to eliminate pain, have stress-free childbirth, get motivated, achieve goals, enhance sports performance, improve at sales, and other life enhancements. One gentleman found that that the light/sound/behavioral repatterning combination ended a five-year battle with chronic hiccups. Another young man came to me with a habitual nose click that even surgery hadn't cured. It stopped during his first session and never came back.

What is the secret to getting these kinds of results?

One of my favorite songs is *Change Your Mind* by Sister Hazel. One of the lines in the song goes, "If you want to be somebody else, if you're tired of fighting battles with yourself . . . change your mind . . ." I love this song because I believe the best way, and sometimes the only way, to make changes in your life is to first change your mind. Because images, beliefs, and values are so deeply rooted in consciousness, changes must happen at the other-than-conscious level before they can manifest in your life. In my experience, the light/sound/behavioral repatterning combination is the quickest and easiest way to change your mind.

If you plant a seed, and know that you are watering and caring for it, you can pretty much sit back, relax, and let it sprout. You wouldn't keep digging up the dirt to see if the seed sprouted, would you? If you did uncover the seed to see if it is sprouting, you would probably stop its growth. I believe that this is what happens when people try to make changes at the conscious level; they set a goal, but then find themselves digging up old images, beliefs, and thought patterns, and end up stopping their growth.

When you relax with light, sound, and behavioral repatterning guiding your conscious mind, you are free to liberate your other-than-conscious mind. Psychologists would say that you are bypassing the critical factor and letting the other-than-conscious mind take over. In other words, you plant the seeds of change, then sit back, relax, and let them sprout.

What are the Best Light & Sound Parameters?

A good choice for a frequency following response program that produces deep relaxation starts at a state of high cortical arousal, a beta frequency of say 15 or 16 Hz. It then ramps down by gradually changing frequency until reaching slow alpha (8 Hz). The frequency should stay there for about seven minutes of the session and then ramp up to a moderate, relaxed alpha (10 Hz). Some programs ramp down into the theta range (4 -7 Hz) in order to achieve a deep other-than-conscious experience. Light and sound combined with positive suggestion, creative visualization, deep relaxation, soothing music, nature sounds, or a combination of these, creates heightened states of awareness.

While there is a wide assortment of relaxation training systems—autogenic (self-produced) training, progressive relaxation, meditation, and biofeedback to name a few—most of these take conscious effort. With the breakthrough of light and sound technology, you don't have to "believe in" or "do" anything. Through the frequency following response, the brain "syncs" to the strobe light and binaural sounds. You are in the experience and don't have to create it.

As an example, if you and I were to go to a secluded beach on a beautiful day while the sunlight reflects off the water and the waves rhythmically pound the sand, and if, while in this environment, we discussed the life improvements you would like to make, chances are good you would enjoy the conversation and accept any advice I might offer. Because of the environment created by this seaside walk, we would be syncing to an alpha state, or about ten cycles per second.

Now if we were to have this same conversation on a bustling street in downtown Manhattan with horns blowing, lights flashing, vendors yelling, and rapid footsteps all around us, we would be syncing to high Beta, or about eighteen cycles per second. The results would be very different. During the city walk, you might get distracted, frustrated, or nervous. In this state, you would be much less open to a conversation about improving your life, and would probably reject any advice I may give, even if it's logical advice. Are you starting to see why brainwaves are so important to our well-being?

What is the Benefit in Achieving the Alpha and Theta States?

Getting out of the fight-or-flight response and into the relaxation response is the best step you can take to overcome the brutal effects of stress. The relaxation response can't happen as long as you generate high beta brainwave activity. Your brainwave activity must dip into alpha, which I refer to as the "intuitive mind," or theta, which I call the "inventive mind."

Because theta is the threshold of sleep, it is best known for lucid dreaming. A person in this state often cannot separate thoughts about his or her awakened state from the lucid dream state. Many believe that theta is the optimum state for creativity and that it's the only place one can make a quantum leap in consciousness. Unfortunately, the theta state is difficult to maintain. When you slip into theta (4-7 Hz), which everyone does at least twice each day (right before falling asleep and just before awakening), and when there are no beta or alpha frequencies mixed with the theta, most people lose consciousness. This is where the frequency following response comes in—it keeps your brain engaged. When people use a light and sound device, they often describe feeling as if their inner experience is more real than the outer experience, which is temporarily suspended.

Researchers might say that these people have entered stage-one sleep, sometimes called the twilight state or the hypnogogic (from the Greek hypnos, meaning sleep, and agnogeus meaning conductor) state. While this is a very healing state, and one that heightens the visualization experience, it was not often used for the purpose of teaching relaxation skills. I believe the results achieved by the thousands of clients who have used the light/sound/behavioral repatterning combination in our franchise programs proves that when a person sees, hears, and experiences the life changes they desire in the alpha and theta states, those changes come to pass in the physical world more quickly and with far less effort.

What are the Benefits of Light and Sound Technology?

Whenever people ask me why I'm so passionate about light and sound technology, I tell them one of my favorite jokes. It goes something like this: One evening a man in a tuxedo rushed up to a street musician and asked, "How do you get to Carnegie Hall?" Without skipping a beat the musician answered, "Practice, man, practice!"

Behavioral repatterning works because it involves mental practice or spaced repetition. In my opinion, there is no faster or easier method for achieving spaced repetition than through the synchronized rhythm of light and sound. The induction into higher brainwave states increases brain activity, while the induction of lower brainwave states reduces hyperactivity and feelings of anxiety.

Brainwave entrainment within alpha states, for example, creates relaxation and a decreased stress response by providing a slower and more relaxed brainwave state. A faster brainwave state, produced by faster flickering of the LED lights, induces a higher brainwave state, and is theorized to enhance brain stimulation and increase cognitive abilities. In many cases, a faster brainwave state can decrease hyperactivity, similar to the paradoxical application of neurostimulant medications such as Ritalin and Dexedrine.

Research showing the efficacy of light and sound technology is not uncommon. Creative visualization and stimulation of brain wave activity are among the most studied areas of psychiatry and psychology. The following results have been demonstrated through numerous studies and in my own experience with thousands of clients:

- *Increased long- and short-term memory*
- *Increased attention span and concentration*
- *Reduction of anxiety and depression*
- *Reduction of medication intake*
- *Increase in right-left visual-spatial integration*
- *Major increase in creativity idea generation*
- *Easier decision making and holistic problem solving*
- *Decrease in migraine or headache frequency and intensity*
- *Reduction in PMS and menopause symptoms*
- *Reduction in insomnia and sleep disorders*
- *Improvement of motivation*

When it comes to losing weight, engaging in behavioral repatterning is one of the most important steps you can take because it works to change your self-image, habits and behaviors. Deep relaxation combined with creative visualization is a powerful tool for creating lasting changes to the eating and lifestlyle habits that ultimately determine your weight and health.

"The only way to discover the limits of the possible is to go beyond them into the impossible."
Arthur C. Clarke

CHAPTER NINETEEN

YOUR METABOLIC REGULATOR: THE THYROID
BY MARK LEWIS, DC

Your Metabolic Regulator: The Thyroid
By Mark Lewis, DC

**What is the importance
of the thyroid in weight loss?**

America is in a health crisis with two out of three Americans being overweight. The National Center for Health Statistics reports that of those Americans that are overweight, more than half are considered obese. While some have hit the gym and others are watching their diets, many are frustrated by their inability to lose weight or keep it off. The losing battle of the bulge has fueled an alarming rise in cardiovascular disease, high blood pressure, diabetes, and cancer.

**What has caused our national health
to spiral out of control?**

One seldom discussed contributor to our country's poor health status is the epidemic of thyroid dysfunction. The Colorado Thyroid Disease Prevalence Study (Arch Intern Med. 2000; 160: 526-534) on over 25,000 participants found that 10% of those studied had an undiagnosed thyroid problem.

This would indicate that 13 million Americans have an abnormal thyroid. According to statistics by the American Association of Clinical Endocrinologists and other medical organizations, approximately 27 million Americans have a thyroid disorder. David Brownstein, M.D., one of our national experts on thyroid disease, states that his own clinical research on over 3000 patients shows our nation's thyroid dysfunction to be closer to 40% and rising.

Chapter 19 | Recognize Hidden Thyroid Problems

The influence of the thyroid on our bodies is pervasive and profound. This butterfly shaped gland, located between our Adam's apple and collar bone, serves as the metabolic regulator for every cell in our body. The hormones produced by the thyroid act to control the metabolism of fats and carbohydrates, absorption of nutrients, strength and rate of our heart beat, blood flow, digestion, respiration, sexual libido and more. In turn, the thyroid exerts an influence on multiple body systems to regulate cholesterol, insulin utilization, immunity, fertility, mental state, body temperature, and to stimulate the proper growth of children.

The primary hormones synthesized by the thyroid are thyroxine (T4) and Triiodothyronine (T3) using the essential amino acid tyrosine and iodine. Iodine is one of the primary components necessary for the creation of thyroid hormones in the body. The thyroid hormones are then converted to their active forms in the liver and kidneys.

The hypothalamus in the brain monitors the blood like a conductor monitoring an orchestra. If the proper amount of thyroid hormone is not being produced, a signal is sent to the anterior pituitary to produce the needed Thyroid Stimulating Hormone (TSH) that is required to bring the system back into harmony.

Assuming the body has a sufficient supply of the necessary nutrients to synthesize the required hormones, the thyroid will respond appropriately to the TSH signal from the pituitary. While 90 percent of the thyroid hormone produced is T4, T3 is significantly more biologically active and exerts the most influence on our body. T3 is produced after T4 drops to the appropriate electron. Calcitonin is also produced by the thyroid and is involved in calcium regulation.

What are the symptoms of an underactive thyroid?

If asked what a person with an underactive thyroid or hypothyroid would look like, you might imagine a person with a goiter. The thyroid swells as it struggles to produce the necessary hormones (T3 and T4) and a visible nodular mass may be observed in the lower throat. While this is one possible and dramatic presentation, there are numerous subtle symptoms of hypothyroidism that are often confused with conditions like chronic fatigue syndrome, fibromyalgia, and autoimmune disorders. In fact, the frequency of hypothyroidism increases with age and is more prominent in women, with 1 out of 5 women over 60 becoming thyroid hormone deficient.

The symptoms of hypothyroidism include:

Difficulty Losing Weight	Hair Loss/Brittle Hair
Muscle Cramps	Fatigue
Feeling Tired	Loss of Outside 1/3 Eyebrows
Puffy Face/Ankles	Constipation
Cold Intolerance	Swollen Tongue
Dry/Itchy Skin	Depression
Cries Often	Morning Headache
Difficulty Swallowing	Goiter
Mental Confusion	Poor Reflexes

The presence of 3 or more of these symptoms would indicate further evaluation using lab testing (blood and urine) to confirm a diagnosis of hypothyroidism. According to Harry O. Eidenier Jr. Ph.D., "a thyroid blood panel without symptoms is useless. 90% of the time the patient is normal on the lab test. If you know the symptoms, numbers become useful." The patient may have a subclinical presentation, which requires a closer evaluation of laboratory values to explain the symptoms.

While Eidenier was working at Brentwood Hospital (an Osteopathic Teaching Facility) in Cleveland Ohio, he regularly performed thyroid panels on whiplash patients upon admission. He noted a significant impairment and hypofunction of the thyroid gland post injury. Eidenier concluded that recovery from neck injuries was critical to the resolution of thyroid dysfunction in these patients. This is supported by Dr. Dan Murphy, who explains that disruption in the sympathetic nervous system caused by a spinal misalignment of the neck can cause "immune system imbalances that are associated with autoimmune diseases such as autoimmune thyroid disease." Manipulation of the neck can be beneficial in treating thyroid dysfunction.

Research indicates that the long term complications of an underactive thyroid can elevate cholesterol, increase cardiovascular and osteoporosis risk, result in infertility, increased 2nd trimester miscarriages, and the impaired IQ of children.

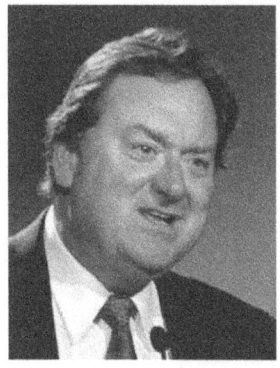

Tim Russert:
Subclinical Hypothyroid

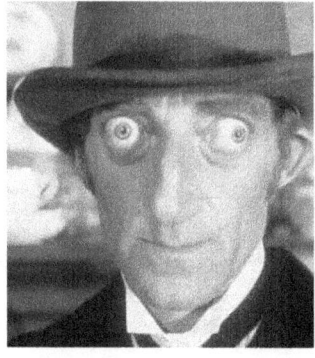

Marty Feldman:
Hyperthyroid (exophthalmoses)

What are the symptoms of an overactive thyroid?

Since the thyroid is directly tied to our metabolic rate, an overproduction of thyroid hormone or hyperthyroidism dramatically speeds up the body metabolism. The heartbeat may rise from 70 beats per minute to 100 beats per minute and become irregular. This creates more stress on our cardiovascular system and can weaken our heart muscle. The symptoms of other health conditions can intensify, along with an increased rate of osteoporosis and digestive problems.

While not as common as hypothyroidism, this condition may signal a more severe health concern. One possible cause of hyperthyroidism is an anterior pituitary tumor that influences the thyroid through TSH. Another would be a dysfunction of the feedback mechanism in the hypothalamus of the brain that monitors the blood stream for the appropriate amount of thyroid hormones. The hypothalamus would produce an excess of Thyrotropic Releasing Hormone (TRH) to stimulate the anterior pituitary to release more TSH. In response to TSH the thyroid would keep producing thyroid hormone and speed up metabolism until it is turned off by the hypothalamus.

One common characteristic of hyperthyroidism is exophthalmoses or "Bug Eyes" and was made famous by actor Marty Feldmen.

Other symptoms include:

Extreme Weight Loss	Muscle Weakness	Hand Tremors
Increased Sweating	Nervousness/ Anxiety	Increased Heart Rate
Heat Intolerance	Extreme Fatigue	Irregular Heart Beat
Diarrhea	Inability to Sleep	Increased Blood Pressure

Another useful method of evaluating thyroid function is the Barnes test. Dr. Broda Barnes noticed a correlation

Chapter 19 | Recognize Hidden Thyroid Problems

between basal body temperature and thyroid dysfunction in the patients he treated. This method has been reported in several clinical studies. Barnes found that the average morning body temperature measured over a five day period immediately upon waking should be between 97.8 and 98.2 degrees. If the temperature was consistently low, then this would be an indication of possible hypothyroidism as the body's metabolism was depressed. The opposite would be true for a patient with hyperthyroism and indicate an increase in metabolism.

Unfortunately, there are many factors (improper technique, poor compliance, low quality thermometer, sleeping under heavy or electric blankets, a restless evening, and fever) that may provide a false reading. Basal body temperature, like any symptom or test, must be considered together with other findings to make a proper diagnosis. Many in the natural healthcare field are taught to treat the patient rather than a specific symptom or test finding. We want to ensure we understand the complete story that the body is trying to relay.

What tests are performed to diagnose a thyroid problem?

After completing a detailed history and exam, blood and urine tests should be ordered to objectively evaluate the thyroid. This allows your doctor to confirm findings and design the appropriate treatment plan. While many simply use TSH to evaluate a thyroid dysfunction this narrow approach has been shown to have limited reliability. According to the British Medical Journal "...treatment should be guided by clinical and metabolic presentation and thyroid hormone concentrations and not by serum TSH concentrations." (BMJ 2003; 326:311-312).

As mentioned previously, TSH is a pituitary hormone that stimulates the thyroid and can often provide a false assessment of the true health of the thyroid. In order to properly evaluate the thyroid, a Free T4 and Free T3 must be ordered to get an accurate measure of their presence in the blood. This will provide a more comprehensive evaluation of thyroid health. If proper hormone levels are present, then the problem may be with the many organs that influence the thyroid like the pituitary, hypothalamus, liver, kidneys, or adrenals.

Reverse T3 should be used to rule out the involvement of the adrenal glands. Under periods of stress (heavy metal toxicity, liver dysfunction or kidney dysfunction) the adrenal glands produce excess cortisol that can disrupt the conversion of T4 to the more active T3. Just like cutting a bad key for a lock, T4 can drop the wrong electron and create a T3 that will not fit the necessary binding sites and is useless. The adrenal glands may also have a negative effect on the hypothalamus and pituitary, which in turn influences the thyroid.

Each member of the orchestra must play their part correctly or it throws off the entire symphony, such is the nature of the endocrine system within which the thyroid exists.

Antibodies may form within the body and attack and destroy the thyroid as in Hashimoto's or Graves disease. Proper thyroid evaluation would also include testing for the presence of thyroid autoantibodies. Poor dietary choices are often named as a significant factor in the development of autoimmune disorders of the thyroid.

Since iodine is a requirement for the synthesis of thyroid hormones, testing for proper iodine levels should be regularly performed. Without iodine or the ability to absorb iodine, the thyroid cannot make hormones. The preferred way to test for iodine levels is using a urinary test kit.

Recommended Lab Test for thyroid

- TSH (Thyroid Stimulating Hormone)
- Free T4 (Thyroxine)
- Free T3 (Triiodothyronine)

- Reverse T3
- Thyroid Autoantibodies
- Urinary Iodine Test

Laboratory tests can only confirm the findings seen in a proper patient history and thorough examination. Tests are prone to false readings and can be misleading if not considered with a full history. In other words, doctors must "treat the patient and not the tests."

What causes thyroid dysfunction and why is it more common?

According to Dr. Mercola, a leading expert in natural and preventive medicine, one reason for an increase in hypothyroid symptoms is our elevated exposure to bromine.

"Bromines are common endocrine disruptors, and are part of the halide family, a group of elements that include fluorine, chlorine, and iodine. What makes it so dangerous is that it competes for the same receptors that capture iodine."

The end result is that as the body's bromine levels rise, iodine levels fall. This not only disrupts the function of the thyroid and it's ability to synthesize hormones, it blocks iodine absorption in every tissue in your body. Some studies suggest that elevated levels of bromine may contribute to an increased risk of cancer and other diseases.

Unfortunately, bromine can be found in significant abundance within our food supply, medication, pool supplies, plastics, fabrics and upholstery, such as:

- Methyl Bromide used as a pesticide on California Strawberries
- Ethylene Dibromide used for soil fumigation and for post harvest treatment
- Brominated Vegetable Oil (BVO) added to citrus

drinks and soda to preserve flavor
- Potassium Bromate added to commercial bakery products, toothpaste and mouthwash
- Polybromo Diphenyl Ethers (PBDEs) in fabric and upholstery as a fire retardant
- Bromine-based hot tub and swimming pool treatment
- Bromine used to manufacture numerous plastic products used daily
- Medications and Anesthetic Agents.

Recognizing the disruptive effect of bromine, the United Kingdom banned the use of bromine in bread. This was followed by Canada and most recently Brazil. Ignoring the growing research, the United States has been slow to identify and address this concern and the negative effects of bromine in baked goods.

Many may remember a popular product from the 1950s called Bromo-Seltzer, that was used as a remedy for hangovers and indigestion. While still on the market, the manufacturers of this product were forced to remove the toxic bromine. Between 1920 and 1960, physician Jorge Flechas reports that there was a 20 percent increase in symptoms of "acute paranoid schizophrenia" due to ingestion of products using bromine that depress the central nervous system (Mercola.com: July 09, 2009; Another Poison Hiding in Your Environment). Symptoms of bromine toxicity consist of the following:

Skin Rashes	*Loss of Appetite*	*Fatigue*
Severe Acne	*Abdominal Pain*	*Metallic Taste*
Cardiac Arrhythmias	*Bleeding Gums*	*Psychological Distress*

Additionally, digestive problems, liver and kidney

dysfunction, and poor protein absorption can alter the production and conversion of thyroid hormone. Personal care products and sunscreens containing Benzalkonium and Benzophenone 2 (BP2) have been shown to negatively affect the thyroid. Pharmacological agents (Antidepressants, Dopamine, Lithium, Glucocorticoids and Tegretol) have also been shown to alter the production of thyroid hormones.

What is the importance of iodine in thyroid dysfunction?

Iodine was discovered by French scientist Bernard Courtiois in the early 1800s and is an essential trace element for life found in ocean foods and soil. The main role of iodine within our body is as a necessary constituent of thyroid hormone. Without iodine, our bodies cannot produce thyroid hormone. The therapeutic application of iodine began in the early 1900s in the Great Lakes region and Midwest where soil erosion and over farming resulted in iodine depletion causing goiters. In 1924 iodized salt was introduced and in four years there was a 75% decrease in goiters.

Iodine was then added to salt and animal feed for the rest of the country. Physicians began to safely and effectively use iodine in the form of Lugol's solution to effectively treat thyroid conditions and related diseases. Iodine was also added to bakery products as an anti-caking agent (Brownstein: Iodine Lecture; August 2009).

Structure of Iodine

After World War II in 1948, a research paper from US Berkley introduced what came to be known as the Wolff-Chaikoff effect, which demonized the use of iodine and falsely claimed that its' use caused hypothyroidism and goiter. The end result of this bombshell was that the United States eventually removed iodine from the food supply in the 1970s. This action was based on poor science and "iodophobia" according to Dr. Guy Abraham, founder of the Iodine Project:

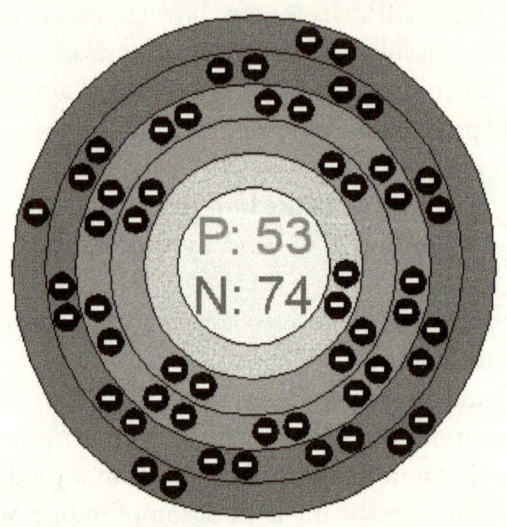

"The demonstration of the Wolff-Chaikoff effect in man remains presumptive. The most effective way to destroy a nation is to remove iodine from the food supply." (Original Internist. 2005 Vol 12: 112-118)

Adding to the controversy, bromine was substituted for iodine in bakery products in the 1970s. Dr. Brownstein feels that "this could be the most asinine act in the history of the food industry." Since the 1970s the National Health and Nutrition Survey reports a 400% increase in moderate to severe iodine deficiency, corresponding with an increased incidence of thyroid illness and cancer. This fear of iodine seems unwarranted when compared to the Japanese who consume 89 times more iodine than Americans (Brownstein: Iodine Lecture; August 2009).

Dr. Mercola states that the Japanese exhibit "reduced rates of many chronic diseases, including the lowest of cancer in the world. The RDA for Iodine in the U.S. is a Meager 150 mcg/day, which pales in comparison with the average daily intake of 13800 mcg/day for the Japanese" (Mercola.com: September 05, 2009; Avoid this if You Want to Keep Your Thyroid Healthy).

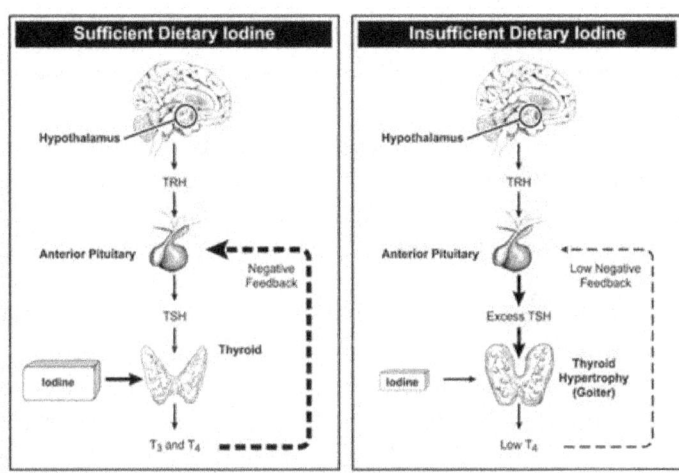

What is the current conventional approach?

The current conventional approach to treating a thyroid condition is through synthetic medication or surgery. A hypothyroid condition is usually managed with synthetic T4 (Synthroid or Levothyroxine) or Synthetic T3 (Cytomel) for life. Unfortunately long term use of this synthetic hormone eventually leads to the thyroid ceasing to function and creates the need for lifelong medication.

A hyperactive thyroid is either removed or destroyed with radioactive iodine and the patient has to again be medicated for life to manage their condition. It is disheartening that many conventional physicians do not take the time to identify the true cause of thyroid problems and its' proper function. A course of conservative care that includes lifestyle changes and the appropriate use of nutritional products have been shown to be extremely effective in reestablishing normal thyroid function.

What is the advantage of using a bioidentical hormone like Armour Thyroid?

Many who suffer from thyroid problems have had their symptoms successfully managed through the use of bioidentical hormones. A bioidentical hormone is a product from an animal or plant source that closely mimics the hormones naturally occurring in the human body. These products cannot be patented and have been extremely effective, so have become a thorn for the pharmaceutical industry.

In particular, Armour Thyroid has been used safely and effectively since the 1890s to treat hypothyroidism.

A 1999 study published in the New England Journal of Medicine that compared the use of Synthroid (Synthetic T4) with Armour Thyroid (natural combination of T3 and T4) found that Armour outperformed Synthroid on every measure. Patients reported improved mood and brain function when taking Armour. Lab tests also confirmed a significant increase in sex hormone-binding globulin over that produced by Synthroid. A few years earlier the FDA echoed these findings when it reported that "...no currently marketed orally administered levothyroxine sodium product [Synthroid] is generally recognized as safe and effective" (Federal Register: August, 14 1997 Vol. 62, Num 157). Over 2 million individuals are currently taking Armour or a generic derivative.

In an odd turn of events, the FDA in September 2009 decided to classify a generic version of Armour as an unapproved new drug. This action has forced two other manufacturers of natural thyroid preparations to suspend production and created three month backorders for the remaining producers. This has angered many physicians who use natural thyroid products including Dr. Johnathan Wright:

"That the FDA should even be thinking of requiring

a new drug approval for a safe, 100 plus year old natural treatment is outrageous" (Healthfreedom.net: September 1, 2009; FDA Attacks Natural Thyroid Millions Depend On). While bioidentical hormones have been used with great success, they are simply replacing a medication with a natural product. The concern with this approach is that it should not be used until a complete course of nutritional therapy, including iodine supplementation and lifestyle modification is completed.

What are some lifestyle recommendations to improve thyroid health?

The goal of any physician should be to encourage the body to function as it was designed to function. This requires patients to seek help from an experienced doctor that will take a detailed approach to uncovering the source of your symptoms and appropriately treat the problem. The conventional approach to treating thyroid dysfunction usually consists of a band-aid approach and simply manages symptoms. There are a number of lifestyle changes that should be incorporated before Synthroid or Armour Thyroid are even considered.

Some dietary changes that can be incorporated include eating organic produce and purchasing organic products as often as possible. Produce should be washed thoroughly to reduce exposure to harmful pesticides. Choosing organic whole-grain bread made with "bromine-free" flour is recommended. Storing food or drinks in plastic containers should be avoided, use glass or ceramic instead. Soft drinks should be avoided and replaced by the consumption of natural non-chlorinated water. Soy isoflavones have been shown to be disruptive to the thyroid and should be avoided.

Choose chemical-free personal care products to avoid exposure to additives that are toxic to the thyroid. An ozone purification system may be substituted in your hot tub and pool to avoid exposure to bromine and chlorine. Opening windows inside buildings and the car can minimize exposure to thyroid toxic products. Cigarettes have also been shown to contain a number of additives that can disrupt thyroid function and should be avoided.

Since it is difficult, at best, to obtain a sufficient amount of our body's required nutrients we must take supplements. A comprehensive review of nutritional research published in the Journal of the American Medical Association concluded that in Western societies "suboptimal vitamin status is associated with many chronic diseases" indicating a need for supplementation (JAMA 2005; 287: 3116-3126). I generally recommend a good quality multi-vitamin, a good B-complex and a balanced essential fatty acid supplement. Patients with thyroid disorders should add iodine supplementation and other nutrients that are indicated by a detailed functional evaluation. Your doctor can be an essential partner in your journey to resolving your thyroid dysfunction and making the proper choices for health.

Dr. Mark Lewis, D.C.
Chiropractic Family Practice Certification
ACA Council on Diagnosis and Internal Disorders
Board Eligible in Clinical Nutrition
The American Clinical Board of Nutrition

Chapter Twenty

The Importance of Water
by Jon Steffins, DC

The Importance of Water
Dr Jon Steffins

As you have read the chapters of this book, you have no doubt been reminded of the wonderful complexity of the human body and how, when given the appropriate opportunity, your body is designed to be a self-regulating self-healing machine. The goal, then, would be to release this healing potential so the body can operate freely within it's innate design and capacity.

To achieve such a worthwhile goal there must be, at the deepest level, a passion to pursue whatever it takes to see that goal become reality. So you continue to educate yourself and your mind transforms itself toward a new way of thinking, a new way of doing, and actually a new way of being. Such significant transformation often requires an open mind and a willingness to consider what you may not have understood before. What follows goes beyond interesting. Open your mind as I take us briefly and simply down a path toward understanding the role of water in the body and how it can and will change your life.

What is The Truth about Water?

"The significant problems we have cannot be solved at the same level of thinking with which we created them." Albert Einstein

The extent of the damage we unintentionally induce in our own bodies is overwhelming. Confusion and misconception are the culprits that lead us down a path of willful, ignorant self-destruction and disease. We think we are safe with our lifestyle and habits. And we are certainly in good company. We follow the whims of good advertising and allow others to dictate what is safe and what is good. For crying out loud, even our healthcare system is numbed by dictatorial commercial interest. We have become fat, dumb and happy; and are as pleased as punch about it. In all of our scientific glory, we chase after treatments and medications emphasizing our paradigm that relief or a better quality of life is just a pill or an injection away.

What Does the Research say?

In the last 25 years, much research has been done that is blazing a distinct trail of understanding that some consider revolutionary. Science is looking at the water molecule with a different set of glasses. What has been theorized, postulated and discovered is nothing short of astounding.

Chemistry has traditionally focused on studying the solutes (that which is dissolved), while viewing what they are dissolved in (the solvent) as nothing more than the "packing material." As research into human biochemistry evolved, that same perspective to understanding was taken. Exhaustive studies have revealed intricate design and order. But an expanded approach to traditional understanding (i.e. different) can be viewed as radical and be categorically discarded. Just as good and intelligent men and women staked their lives and reputations on the 'knowledge' that the earth was flat… an enlarged perspective of the role of the water molecule is met with both resistance and hope. Throw into the mix the vast industrial machine that has evolved pursuing a particular responsible or patentable substance to treat disease or manipulate body chemistry and the challenge in a paradigm shift is pretty obvious. Over the years, very little connection between hydration and disease has been made. Some have made it their life's work to validate that connection.

It would be simplistic to make the claim that any one thing is a "cure all" in the same way that it would be foolish to dismiss all medication as inappropriate or current research as misguided. A fresh perspective, however, throws light on an interesting lowest common denominator approach. The focus of that perspective being the dominant metabolic role of water in the body, the hydroelectric nature of water as it crosses the cell membrane, and the relationship of water (dehydration) to conditions, symptoms, and disease. As research validates this approach, water becomes a key player in dealing with our toxic acidic bodies as well as the current obesity epidemic.

Water is energy

The undisputed fact is that all known forms of life depend on water. Without water the metabolic processes would cease to exist. Water is central to acid-base neutrality and enzyme function. The body has a terrifically intricate water management or regulation system and prioritizes where available water resources go. At the end of the day, that regulatory system relates directly to energy supply and demand. In other words, the body calls for water when energy supply must be replenished. It is the energy need of the body that dictates the water regulation system.

There also exists, as a result of the aging process (past the age of twenty), a progressive inability to recognize the need to take on water, i.e. the thirst mechanism. So as we age, even when our bodies are thirsty, we may not get the message – or worse, the message we get is interpreted incorrectly. Even what we know as "dry mouth" is treated as an inadequate measuring stick as the primary indicator of thirst.

When the body is fully hydrated, blood is about 94 percent water. Most of the cells of the body ideally contain about 75 percent water. The brain equates to $1/50^{th}$ of total body weight with roughly nine trillion nerve cells. Brain cells are 85% water so it is easy to deduce why 20 percent of the blood supply is allocated to the brain. Your body must supply the brain's constant demand for energy. The brain must stay hydrated.

The late Dr. F. Batmanghelidj contended strongly that in addition to metabolized food (sugar), the brain depends on its water supply for hydroelectric energy. Free water flow across the membranes of our cells generates energy that is utilized to replenish and restore spent energy stockpiles. When the cells use up their energy stores, the message to produce more is generated. The thirst/hunger mechanism is triggered to bring fuel on board. Since water intake depends on the sensation of thirst, which decreases as we age, an incipient and gradually establishing chronic dehydration will lead to a symptom producing physiological state of the human body. Our body cries out for water and we do not recognize it.

Are You Energy Bankrupt?

On top of not realizing we are thirsty, consider how we have changed as a culture over the past 50 years. In today's world, a functionally abnormal use of our bodies is more common than not. People have become inactive, highly stressed couch potatoes. So we live in an energy demanding, chronically dehydrated, sedentary world. Is it any wonder that we are fatigued and fat? Little did we know how important a piece of the puzzle our little water molecule is.

Let's connect the water dots.

1. Stress, fatigue and hydration are intimately associated as water availability, or hydration, *directly* relates to the level of energy production on the cellular level;
2. By and large, we are less physically active; so in spite of having fat energy stores on board, the biochemical events required to tap into that energy do not take place so it goes unused. The body cries out for energy using a thirst mechanism that apparently deprograms itself as we age. So instead of water intake, we eat (in increasing portions to supply demand). We fail to feed our thirst.
3. We are chronically toxic and acidic (due to diet, lifestyle, and medication) which uses up more energy, dehydrates even further, and engages the self-preservation mechanism of surrounding the toxins in fat and storing it out of circulation.
4. And finally, and most damaging, we incorrectly accept the notion that fluid intake is the same as water intake. Though our drinks *contain* water they, more often than not, actually contribute to and lead to dehydration. We fall prey to tasty addictive products that lead us ever onward toward energy bankruptcy.

This cycle takes us ever deeper into the territory of unwanted weight gain.

Mundane to Exotic

How do you make the decision to reverse the trend? Understand first, your body is not sick. It is thirsty. To function properly, the body requires between one and seven liters of water per day to avoid dehydration. Depending on temperature, activity levels, humidity and other factors like moisture content of food intake, most agree that 6 to 8 glasses of water (around 2 liters) is the ***minimum*** to maintain proper hydration. A good way to determine the least amount of water you need daily is to take your weight and divide by two and then drink that many ounces. For example, if you weigh 192 pounds you would drink 96 ounces--six 16-ounce glasses as a minimum--of plain, pure **water**!

I often am asked why we should drink water as opposed to the pleasing, taste enhanced beverages that are hyped and marketed as fine, fulfilling and fun! My answer is simple. Many of our healthcare challenges can be traced directly to what we drink. To equate drinking a glass water to drinking a can of some beverage is a fundamental misunderstanding. Think about it. Our most popular beverages contain ingredients that alter the body's chemistry, exhaust energy supply, and are addicting. A quick glance at the so-called diet drinks uncovers even more damaging truth. Diet beverages introduce artificial sweeteners into the system, which in short, prompts the liver to stop manufacturing sugar from raw materials and to begin storing sugar. When the sugar that was promised through the taste buds is nowhere to be found, the sensation of hunger is produced to find food to deliver on the promise of energy. Here we get on that weight gain merry-go-round again. The damage we do to our bodies by habitual consumption of manufactured beverages cannot be overemphasized and would be the impetus for much further discussion.

Taking a quick look at some or our other popular beverages, it is well known that alcoholic beverages dehydrate the body. In this area, moderation is key. Milk should be treated as a food. Cow's milk is made to be drunk by cow babies to help them grow quickly. There is controversy over reconstituted pulpless juices… and on and on. We could write volumes on the so-called energy drinks. Once again, realize that fluid intake does not compare to water intake.

Twenty first century options of "drinking water" range from the mundane to the exotic. The shelves at the grocery stores are lined with choices. The bottom line as to the choice of what water to drink must then be determined by what are the expected gains.

Though bacteriologically safe in most cases, it is not advisable to drink city tap water due to the water recycling and purification process. Natural spring water is a better option; but ground water contamination from detergents, farm chemicals and even radiation must be considered when making this choice. Commercially produced drinking water from city water supplies--with "added minerals for taste"-- is another good choice over tap water and it is readily available. A better choice even than the ones above is distilled water; but that too, has had its share of controversy. The concern has been expressed that distilled water may leach valuable minerals from the body. It does, however produce a negative ion reaction in the system and negative ions are alkaline forming, which attracts positively charged acid waste products and flushes them toward the elimination channels. Even though most distilled water tests acidic due to its negative charge, a more alkaline internal environment is created in the body when distilled water is consumed.

Water... No Additives needed

Another option for drinking water comes from a technology developed through Japanese research over the last half of the Twentieth century. It is known as electronically restructured alkaline water. There are many health claims from all around the world from using this water as a part of a weight loss/weight management protocol. Water, plain water, is wonderful. Throw in a little lemon for additional alkalinity and it is a delightful beverage. And now, with filtered electrolyzed ionized water, our little H_2O molecule has gone from simple solvent to antimicrobial agent to use as a medical treatment of disease in many countries.

Of the many options that are available, electronically restructured alkaline water would arguably be the optimum choice for the greatest gain in re-hydrating the body. This type of water can now be produced with a special unit right at your own sink. The water processed through one of these units actually is reconfigured to a lighter simpler form that is more absorbable in the body. Not only do you get a product that is beneficial electrically, restructured water alkalizes by displacing acids and replacing alkalines...and that is beneficial to life, health, and wellness.

Knowledge is the beginning of wisdom.

The importance of water is undeniable. Understanding of the role of water in the production of energy in the body is revolutionary. The discovery of the connection between dehydration and weight gain is liberating. Knowing the truth about the self-imposed destructive addictive nature of manufactured beverages and their link to obesity is empowering. Good water is key. Ionized alkaline water is optimal for maximum energy and hydration.

Light obeyed increases light. Light rejected increases night. And there is no night so dark as that which is self imposed.

Six Tips to Drinking More water:

1. Understand that chances are you are dehydrated, which leads to lowered energy and increased hunger;
2. Understand you need to detoxify and de-acidify as you lose weight;
3. Understand alkaline water is your beverage of choice for optimal results;
4. Understand lifestyle change regarding nutrition and exercise is imperative;
5. Understand that you are not alone, and
6. Understand that your HealthSource Doctors are uniquely positioned to help you every step of the way on your journey to greater quality of life and health.

Drink water, and live well. Use optimal water and change your life. But remember, it is only when passion evolves to performance; when knowledge leads from understanding to implementation; when desire for change outweighs the discomfort inherent in change that any truth has the power to set you free.

CHAPTER TWENTY-ONE

Exercise and Weight Loss
by Jeff Wisdo, DC

Exercise and Weight Loss
Jeff Wisdo

How many times have you heard about the next greatest diet where you can lose weight – even with no exercise! Sounds great, doesn't it? The truth is that we can all lose weight if we burn more calories than we consume over any given period of time. It really is that simple! The problem for most people is maintaining the weight loss for years. In this chapter you will learn how exercise can help you lose weight, maintain it for life and all of the other positive effects that exercise can have on your health. Also, we will discover what the best exercises for weight loss are; and how to go about starting your new exercise program for life!

The role of exercise in overall health

All through this book, you have read about the makeup of food and how it affects your weight, good versus bad carbohydrates, and many other important topics concerning long-lasting weight loss and health. There may be no more important topic in this book for long term weight loss and overall health than exercise. Yes, you read that correctly. There is nothing else that will help you lose the weight and keep it off than a good, sustainable, lifelong exercise program. This lifelong exercise program doesn't necessarily mean an hour at the gym six days a week for the rest of your life. Nor does it mean you need to look like you are entering the local bodybuilding competition. We will describe what we mean later, but first let's look at the effect exercise has on our bodies.

The benefits of exercise go way beyond weight loss. People who exercise regularly have both physical and psychological benefits. Overall, they will be healthier for longer. One of the biggest benefits of exercise is the reduced risk of developing cardiovascular disease. In a study published in *The New England Journal of Medicine,* the researchers followed over 70,000 female nurses over a period of eight years. All were measured on the amount of exercise that they performed over the study time.

This exercise varied from vigorous exercise to simple walking to little or no exercise. The study found that women who either exercise vigorously for 1.5 hours per week or walked briskly for 3 hours per week had reduced their risk of cardiovascular disease by 30 to 40 percent. The study also found that those women who previously had a sedentary lifestyle and started a moderate exercise program decreased their risk for developing cardiovascular disease.[1]

Other physical benefits of exercise include lower cholesterol, decreased risk of diabetes, lower blood pressure, lower heart rate, increased muscle mass, increased bone density; thus decreasing the occurrence of osteoporosis, increased strength of ligaments and tendons while increasing flexibility. Together this reduces the risk of injuries due to slips and falls--to name just a few.

---

[1] A prospective study of walking as compared with vigorous exercise in the prevention of coronary heart disease in women. Manson JE, Hu FB, Rich-Edwards JW, Colditz GA, Stampfer MJ, Willett WC, Speizer FE, Hennekens CH. N Engl J Med. 1999 Aug 26;341(9):650-8.

Regular exercise has also been shown to be good for our mental health.

There have been hundreds of studies that show a reduction in symptoms of both anxiety and depression with regular exercise. With all of the benefits of exercise both physically and mentally, what are the drawbacks? The simple answer is there are none! As described previously, walking 30 minutes a day is good for almost every organ in your body--as well as putting you in a good mood.

The role of exercise in weight loss

Will exercise help me lose weight and keep it off? YES. Ultimately, losing weight is about consuming fewer calories than we expend over a period of time--one day, one week, one month or one year. The more we exercise, the more calories we burn, the more weight we lose over that period of time. But more importantly than simply exercising is the type of exercise we do and its effect on our body and our basal metabolic rate.

Basal metabolic rate (BMR) is defined as the amount of energy (calories) our body needs to function at rest. This includes the energy needed by our body's organs to continue to function--the heart, liver, brain, skin, muscles and everything else. We also know that our BMR decreases with age and with muscle mass.

There are some very complex formulas to help estimate this number for individuals, but these generally do not take into account lean body mass or other factors that can cause this to deviate. Many local health clubs and gyms have more elaborate equipment to measure this if you are interested.

Ultimately, the more skeletal muscle mass, the higher the BMR and the more calories that someone burns at rest. With all of that being said, one of the goals of any long term weight loss exercise program should be to burn calories while at the same time increasing lean (skeletal) muscle mass.

What are the best exercises for me to help with my weight loss?

Whenever we start an exercise program, the most important thing is to choose an exercise that you will enjoy long term. If you don't enjoy swimming, then joining your local YMCA so that you can swim laps is probably not a good plan. You will want to pick something that you enjoy and can easily fit into your schedule.

There are so many exercise programs and DVDs on the market to choose from if that is what interests you. You can join a gym, go to the local sporting goods store and buy an elliptical machine or treadmill, buy a pair of walking shoes. The options are limitless, but the most important thing is make it something that it is easy to do every day as you will need to exercise at least 30 minutes per day. Below is a chart of calories burned for various activities. These numbers are only estimates and vary depending on intensity, weight, level of physical fitness and other factors.

Activity (one-hour duration)	Weight of person and calories burned		
	160 pounds	200	240
Aerobics, high impact	511	637	763
Aerobics, low impact	365	455	545
Aerobics, water	292	364	436
Backpacking	511	637	763
Basketball game	584	728	872
Bicycling, < 10 mph, leisure	292	364	436
Bowling	219	273	327
Canoeing	256	319	382
Dancing, ballroom	219	273	327
Football, touch, flag, general	584	728	872
Golfing, carrying clubs	329	410	491
Hiking	438	546	654
Ice skating	511	637	763
Jogging, 5 mph	584	728	872
Racquetball, casual, general	511	637	763
Rollerblading	913	1,138	1,363
Rope jumping	730	910	1,090
Rowing, stationary	511	637	763
Running, 8 mph	986	1,229	1,472
Skiing, cross-country	511	637	763
Skiing, downhill	365	455	545
Skiing, water	438	546	654
Softball or baseball	365	455	545
Stair treadmill	657	819	981
Swimming, laps	511	637	763
Tae kwon do	730	910	1,090
Tai chi	292	364	436
Tennis, singles	584	728	872
Volleyball	292	364	436
Walking, 2 mph	183	228	273
Walking, 3.5 mph	277	346	414
Weightlifting, free weight, Nautilus or universal type	219	273	327

Source: Ainsworth BE, Haskell WL, Whitt MC, Irwin ML, Swartz AM, Strath SJ, O'Brien, WL, Bassett DR Jr, Schmitz KH, Emplaincourt PO, Jacobs DR Jr, Leon AS. Compendium of physical activities: an update of activity codes and MET intensities. Med Sci Sports Exerc. 2000 Sep;32(9 Suppl):S498-504.

Ideally, we would like to burn fat tissue as a result of our exercising. This has much more to do with the intensity of the exercise. Generally speaking, fat burning exercises are those that are long duration with a steady pace and involve the greatest number of muscles. Exercises in this category are walking, running, elliptical machine, swimming, or biking.

Typically, these activities can be performed for extended periods of time with breaks to catch your breath. The other types of exercise that would typically burn more sugars are those that have a quick burst of activity then a rest period. Exercise in this category would be basketball, tennis, and racquetball. This is not to say that playing tennis or basketball is not advised, but you will generally burn more sugars and less fat. However, ultimately, the goal is to burn more calories doing something that you enjoy.

The other part of your weight loss exercise program needs to be some type of resistance training in order to build lean muscle mass. This can be done at the gym with free weights or machines. You can also buy resistance bands at a sporting goods store or the sports department at your local Wal-Mart or Target. Resistance training can include a home regiment of push-ups, sit-ups and pull-ups. The goal is to increase your muscle mass so that your BMR increases. You don't need to look like an NFL linebacker, but increasing your muscle mass will help in keeping off that weight long term.

Walking - The Perfect Weight Loss Exercise

Walking is the perfect exercise for losing weight. It is easy to start, you can do it anywhere and most of us have been doing it since we were infant. Walking is a sustained exercise that will burn fat. The only equipment that you will need is a good pair of walking or athletic shoes.

You can walk anywhere – at home, on vacation, during your lunch break at work – and anytime – before you go to work, work breaks, after work, weekdays and weekends. You can do it by yourself. You can find a partner to walk with such as a spouse, kids, parents, friends, family or dog. Walking is an all purpose, weight burning machine that will give you all of the benefits of exercise that we mentioned earlier. Plus you can start at any time no matter your current fitness level.

I suggest this to be the exercise of choice for anyone starting a weight loss program. It is cheap and effective. Whenever starting a new program, start slowly. For some, this may mean walking around the block for the first week. For others, it can be walking 30 minutes. Do not overexert yourself as this will cause sore muscles and can lead to injuries.

Before walking, make sure you stretch and warm up your body. This can be done with simple stretches such as touching your toes, doing ankle circles and trunk rotations. As with any exercise, make sure that you have good posture and technique. Keep your head looking forward with your shoulders relaxed and your arms swinging comfortably at your side. During your walks, you should be able to hold a conversation. If you can't hold a conversation, you are walking too fast. If you are breathing like you do at rest, walk faster.

Drink plenty of water before, during and after any exercising. The end goal should be walking briskly (4 miles per hour) 30 minutes per day 6 days a week within 10 weeks.

For most people, this simple exercise program would increase their health way beyond any weight loss benefits.

My Walking Story

I confess, I am a walker. I love it. I hate to run, but I know that I need a weight bearing exercise to help me control my weight, but also to improve my health as well. I am also a very goal oriented person, so just walking for me is not really a whole lot of fun.

Yes, I can walk with my iPhone and listen to music or talk to people, but I always need a challenge. For my walking, I challenge myself to walking marathons. 26.2 miles of walking. This challenge has helped me lose 136 pounds.

When I started, I was not able to walk more than three or four miles, but ended with all 26.2. Walking allows me to clear my head, feel better and most importantly improve my life through sustained weight loss and healthy habits.

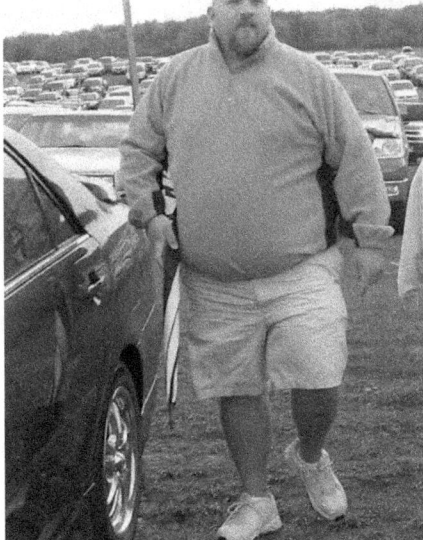

Just Do It!

In the end, you can lose weight just by dieting. Adding an exercise program is essential to keeping the weight off for life--not to mention the benefits of exercise for your health, both physically and mentally. No matter if you decide to walk, play basketball, swim, or ride a bike, just start doing something that you enjoy. Make sure that it easily fits into your lifestyle. No one can exercise for you, so JUST DO IT!

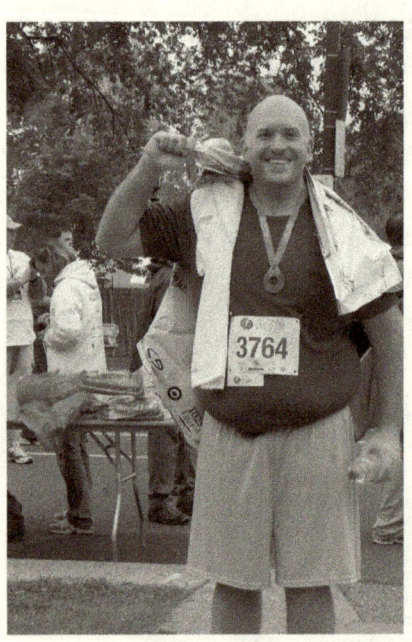

CHAPTER TWENTY-TWO

ADDITIONAL RESOURCES

Chapter One: The Acid/Base Balance
by Richard Kearns, DC

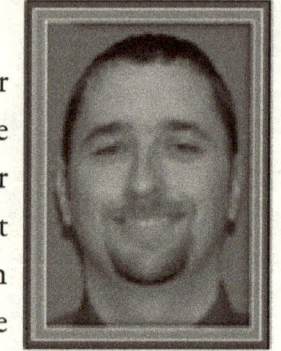

Dr. Kearns, as a chiropractor and father, knows the importance of keeping children and their families subluxation free to prevent nervous system interference through effective, gentle chiropractic care. He graduated from Youngstown State University in 1999 and Palmer College of Chiropractic in 2004. He has had additional post graduate training in Flexion Distraction and spinal decompression.

Dr. Kearns has given presentations to Kid's Day America and other civic organizations. His topics of presentation include "Its your Future, Be there Healthy", nutrition, back pain, disc herniations, and spinal decompression. His office is located in Avon, Ohio and offers caring and compassionate care for their chiropractic patients.

Chapter Two:
Oxygenating the Body – The Lymphatic System
by Chad Young, DC

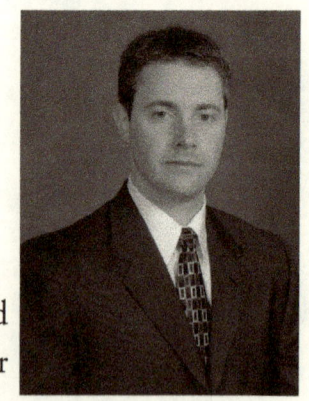

Dr. Chad Young has lived and practiced in Paducah, Kentucky for

7 years. He has earned a bachelor's degree in Human Biology, a Doctorate of Chiropractic, and completed post graduate studies in nutrition. If Dr. Young isn't helping people at his chiropractic office or at his fitness club you can usually find him spending time with his wife Stacy and sons Jacob and Tyler.

Chapter Three: Detoxifying the Body and Weight Loss
by Joseph Hayes, DC

Dr. Hayes received his doctorate in Chiropractic from the Palmer College of Chiropractic in 1997. He is licensed by the National Board of Chiropractic Examiners for Parts I, II, III and IV in the state of Maine. His professional associations include the Christian Chiropractor's Association, the Palmer Alumni Foundation and the Maine Chiropractic Association.

Dr. Hayes has also been certified in many varied techniques including extremity adjusting, cox lumbar flexion distraction technique, Logan basic technique, Physiotherapy, Rehabilitation of acute and chronic conditions, certification in whiplash and brain traumatology, the Graston Technique and cold laser techniques. His Health Source Chiropractic practice is in Portland, Maine.

Chapter Four: Feeding the Body -- Body Chemistry
by Amanda Borre, DC

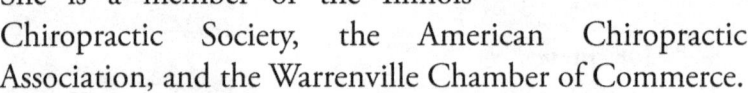

Dr. Borre graduated from the Southern Illinois University and Logan College of Chiropractic. Her post graduate training includes hours for acupuncture, spinal decompression, pain management, pain management and nutrition. She is a member of the Illinois Chiropractic Society, the American Chiropractic Association, and the Warrenville Chamber of Commerce.

Dr. Borre has given presentations to many civic groups and organizations including Weight Watchers. She has spoken on many topics such as "Its Your Future, Be There Healthy", nutrition, back pain, spinal decompression and industrial safety and health.

Dr. Borre's clinic is in Warrenville, Illinois. They offer chiropractic, progressive rehabilitation, acupuncture and decompression therapy. She is a busy mother of two children and is a firm believer in getting and staying healthy.

Chapter Five: Dispelling the Myths – Protein
By Frank Dachtler, DC

Dr. Frank Dachtler received his B.A. in Chemistry and Psychology from Case Western Reserve University. After working as a chemist for the U.S. EPA emergency technical assistance team, he attended Cleveland Chiropractic College in Kansas City, where he graduated Magna

Cum Laude in 1998. After graduation, Dr. Dachtler opened his first practice in Bedford, Ohio.

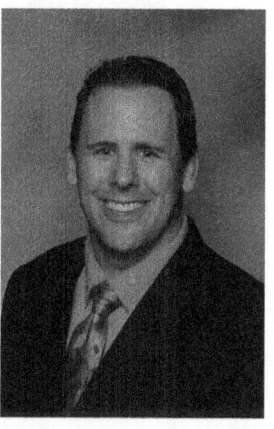

He built a successful business and decided to join HealthSource in April of 2006, in order to expand his office. Since that time, he has opened two additional clinics in Norton and South Toledo, Ohio, both as HealthSource franchises. He brings to the team an extensive knowledge of marketing and its principles, as well as an understanding of the HealthSource model from a practical standpoint.

Chapter Six: Sugar Awareness
by Brandon Pettke, DC

Over the years, Dr. Pettke has taken care of thousands of patients. He has treated all walks of life including government employees, managers, CEOs, children and athletes of all kinds from student to amateur to professional. He is an avid sports fan and plays many sports. He lives in Forth Worth, Texas with his wife and kids.

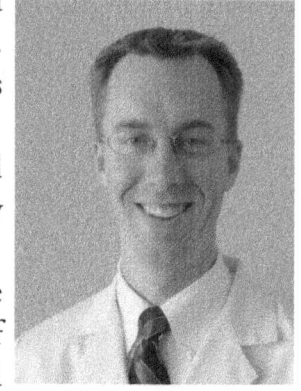

Dr. Pettke's educational experience began at the University of Texas at Austin.

He continued his graduate work at Parker College of Chiropractic where he graduated in 2003. He received a Bachelor of Science in Anatomy and a Doctorate in Chiropractic Medicine. He was distinguished by being on the Dean's Honor Roll. He is a member of the American Chiropractic Association and the Texas Chiropractic Association.

Dr. Pettke's post graduate studies include the topics of carpal tunnel syndrome, low level laser therapy, neurology, nutrition, pathomechanics of radiculopathy, post injury rehabilitation, spinal decompression therapy, spinal rehabilitation and x-ray. He has given seminars on back pain, carpal tunnel, fibromyalgia, headaches, neck pain, nutrition, plantar fasciitis and weight loss.

Chapter Seven: Importance of Fiber in Weight Loss and Health
by Jessi Rezac, BS

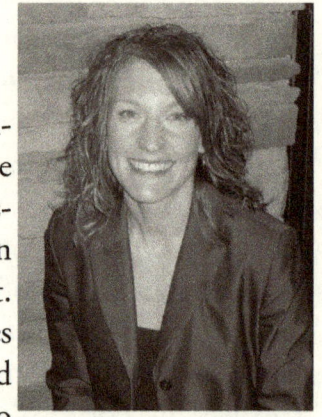

Jessica Rezac is a nutritionist based in Armstrong, IA. She graduated in 2003 with her Master's Degree in Human Nutrition from the University of Bridgeport. In her current role, Jessica educates patients on how to lose weight and improve their diet and lifestyle to achieve their highest level of health. These duties combine with her special training in FirstLine Therapy (therapeutic lifestyle changes). She also speaks on a variety of topics including weight loss, ADD/ADHD, arthritis, fibromyalgia, menopause, and infertility.

Jessica lives in Armstrong with her husband, Dr. Corey Rezac, DC, their three children, and two dogs.

When not working, Jessica likes to play with her kids, cook, workout, and relax with her husband. Jessica can be reached at healthsource@iowatelecom.net.

Chapter Eight: The Roll of Enzymes in Health and Weight Loss
by Mason Orth, DC

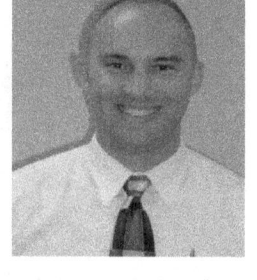

Dr. Orth has a Health Source Chiropractic practice located in Fargo, North Dakota. He graduated from Minnesota State University in 1993 and from Northwestern Health Sciences University in 1999. He is a member of the American Chiropractic Society and the North Dakota Chiropractic Association.

His post graduate training includes work in impairment rating, whiplash and trauma, pain management, non surgical spinal decompression, radiology, balance disorders and nutrition.

Dr. Orth is also considered a sports medicine specialist. In addition to providing care to local student athletes and coaches he has also treated many professional and amateur atheletes.

His speaker credentials include topics such as arthritis, osteoporosis, fibromyalgia, nutrition and supplementation, carpal tunnel syndrome, balance disorders, dizziness, back pain, diabetes, cardiovascular health, cancer prevention, wellness and weight loss.

Chapter Nine: the Immune System and Weight Loss
by Michael J. Porter, BS

Michael J. Porter was Director of Nutrition for the Positive Changes franchise for more than fourteen years. In that time, Michael developed the 21 Steps to Better Health and Nutrition, which was designed specifically for weight-loss clients and has since helped thousands to lose weight and improve their health. This program enhances the knowledge of the client with cutting-edge nutritional information; it is an all-around health and wellness learning series that can be used by any one to help promote optimum health.

Michael started researching health and nutrition in 1974 when he uncovered his own food sensitivities and transformed his health through better nutrition. He has since been sharing his knowledge with others through special reports, video and audio recorded messages, magazine and newsletter articles, and on websites and blogs. The breadth and depth of his health and nutrition knowledge is unparalleled, which is why he is a popular guest on radio shows. Michael received his BS from Quantum University in Hawaii.

Chapter Ten: Changing Your Beliefs About Weight Loss
by Patrick K. Porter, Ph.D.

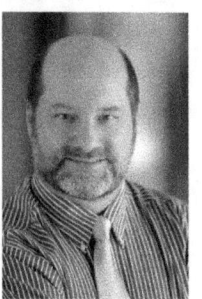

Patrick K. Porter, Ph.D. is an award-winning author, entrepreneur, and experienced speaker. With 24 years of experience operating the largest self-help franchise, he has become a highly sought-after expert within the personal improvement industry. He is the Creator of the ZenFrames, Behavioral Repatterning Device (BRD) which is used by the HealthSource doctors to help people overcome stress and insomnia, lose weight, stop smoking, manage pain, accelerate learning, and much more.

Previously, he founded Positive Changes, the world's largest franchise network of lifestyle improvement centers. Dr. Porter's successes were featured in *The Wall Street Journal, BusinessWeek, People, Entrepreneur,* and *INC,* as well as ABC, NBC, CBS, and the Discovery Channel.

He is the author of the bestselling book, *Awaken the Genius, Mind Technology for the 21st Century,* which was awarded "Best How-To Book of 1994" by the North American Book Dealers Exchange. He is also author of *Discover the Language of the Mind,* and *Six Secrets of G.E.N.I.U.S.* Dr. Porter has produced an arsenal of more than 300 audio-recorded motivational programs and creative visualization processes, and has sold more than three million books and recordings worldwide. The material from this chapter has been adapted from his book, *Thrive In Overdrive, How to Navigate Your Overloaded Lifestyle.*

Chapter Eleven:
Fats Your Body Needs and Why – Essential Fatty Acids
by Chris Tomshack, DC

Dr. Chris Tomshack is the founder and CEO of HealthSource Chiropractic and Progressive Rehab. After graduating with honors from Ohio University with a Bachelor's of Business Administration, he was also commissioned an officer in the United States Air Force, graduating top in his ROTC class. He then continued his study at the University of Toledo, where he was in the MBA program as well as serving as a teaching assistant in the marketing department. Dr. Tomshack then enrolled in Palmer College of Chiropractic, where he graduated Summa Cum Laude. After graduation, Dr. Tomshack immediately opened his practice in Vermilion, Ohio. Practice growth came slow at first, finally reaching the point where Dr. Tomshack had the busiest practice around. He then retired from active practice at age 37 and began building multiple offices, opening three more successful practices. Many of the practice and business principles he introduced into his clinics came from his relentless study of other industries, always looking for ways to improve the way a practice should be run.

Realizing that he and his team had put together some of the most progressive treatment protocols and business systems ever introduced into chiropractic, he began the steps of building a true franchise for other chiropractors. Dr. Tomshack launched HealthSource Chiropractic and Progressive rehab in April of 2006, and in a short time they have become the fastest growing franchise business and opportunity in chiropractic today, helping to build many successful and thriving practices all across the country.

Chapter Twelve: Reversing the Aging Process and Weight Loss
by Jeremy Busch, DC

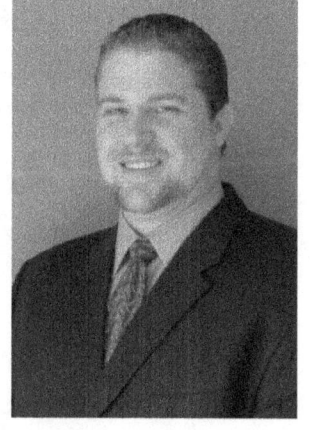

Dr. Busch is not only a doctor of chiropractic but also a Board Certified Chiropractic Sports Physician, a Certified Strength and Conditioning Specialist, and a Certified Hypnotherapist. His educational training includes a degree from Michigan State University in 1999, the National University of Health Sciences in 2006 and the Graduate Hospital in Philadelphia, PA, also in 2006. His post graduate training includes hours in sports injuries and rehabilitation, hypnotherapy, acupuncture and strength training and conditioning.

He is a member of the Christian Chiropractic Association, the Virginia Chiropractic Association, The American Chiropractic Association, American Chiropractic Sports Physicians and several others. He has also received training in kinesiotaping, extremity injuries and rehabilitation, nutrition, botanicals, homeopathy, pain management, and Chi Running and Chi walking.

Dr. Busch has honored several organizations by

sharing his knowledge including Virginia Tech University, Radford University, the Radford City Chamber of Commerce and the YMCA. He speaks on a variety of topics including peak performance, golf performance, osteoporosis, arthritis, fibromyalgia, nutrition, weight loss, exercise, back pain, injury, balance disorders and industrial health and safety.

Dr. Busch's practice is located in Front Royal, Virginia and includes the care of many local student athletes and coaches as well as professional and amateur athletes, dance companies and musicians.

Chapter Thirteen: Metabolism -- Natural Nutrients vs. Stimulants
by Andy Nelson, DC

Dr. Nelson received his undergraduate degree from Yavapai College in basic sciences and his chiropractic training from the Texas Chiropractic College. He has been in private practice for nine years focusing on full scope chiropractic and progressive rehabilitation including weight loss and nutrition.

Dr. Nelson received post graduate training in acupuncture, chiropractic biophysics, advanced clinical nutrition, physical medicine and rehabilitation. He is a board certified chiropractic physician and a Biocranial Institute certified practitioner.

He has been married for twenty five years and is

a proud father and grandfather. He is a CTM lecturer, a Competent Toastmaster, Missionary, Volunteer leader for the Boy Scouts of America, competitive 10K runner and exercise enthusiast including playing racquetball, camping, fishing and hiking. His Health Source Chiropractic Clinic is located in Prescott, Arizona

Chapter Fourteen: Breaking Through Plateaus: Understanding Plateaus in Weight Loss
by Jim Hoven, DC

Dr. Hoven attended Colorado State University and then went on to receive his Doctorate of Chiropractic at Logan College of Chiropractic. Since that time, Dr. Hoven has served the health care industry as a provider, an educator, and a trainer in many different organizations.

Through extensive lecturing and community involvement, he has built several successful chiropractic practices throughout the Denver area and has been requested to lecture at numerous business, civic, and governmental events. More recently, Dr. Hoven has traveled the country consulting with medical clinics on documentation and coding issues related to physical medicine procedures.

He currently serves Health Source members through franchise development and training.

Chapter Fifteen: Eating a Balanced Meal
by Michele Askar, DC

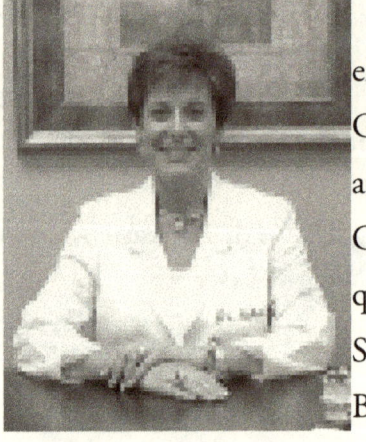

Dr. Askar received her bachelor's of science degree from Gannon University. She then attended the Life Chiropractic College in Georgia and subsequently opened her own Health Source Chiropractic clinic in Beaver County, Pennsylvania utilizing the most updated techniques in progressive rehabilitation and decompression technology for her patients who suffer from chronic back and neck pain. Dr. Askar also offers CBP adjusting as well as weight loss programs within her practice. She specializes in treating carpal tunnel and fibromyalgia.

Dr. Askar decided on chiropractic as a career because of her experiences with the health care field within her family. She felt there had to be a better way to health than treating patients as guinea pigs. She studied every technique available and attended many extra seminars to learn what she could about health and wellness and now, fifteen years later, her patients in Pennsylvania are benefitting from her personal compassion and knowledge.

Chapter Sixteen: How Stress Affects Weight Loss
by Brady Schuyler, DC

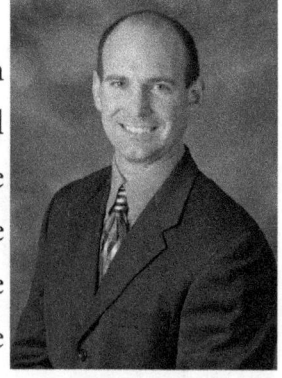

Dr. Schuyler believes in treating each patient as an individual person, not a condition. He uses the highest quality care, which is possible through his training received at the University of Wisconsin-La Crosse in 1997 and the National University of Health Science in 2001. His post graduate training includes training for x-ray, acupuncture, whiplash and trauma, pain management, nutrition, carpal tunnel syndrome, and spinal decompression. He is also a muscle activation specialist (M.A.T).

Dr. Schuyler is a member of the American Chiropractic Association and has participated in many speaking engagements to a variety of audiences including The International Administration of Administrative Professionals. His topics have included a myriad of subjects such as golf performance, nutrition, fibromyalgia, osteoporosis, arthritis and stress management.

Dr. Schuyler's Health Source Clinic is located in Plainfield, Illinois.

Chapter Seventeen: Understanding the Neurotransmitters and Hormones that Affect Weight Control
by Steven Troeger, DC & Deborah L. Troeger, B.S., M.A., C.C.H.T.

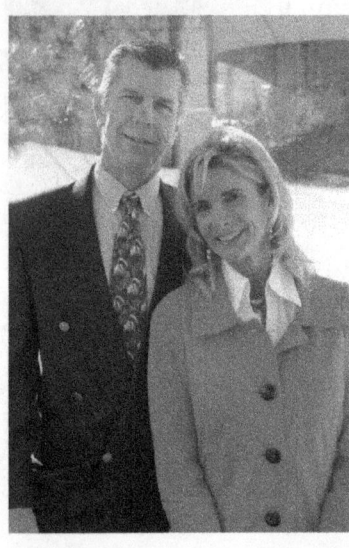

Dr. Troeger is a graduate of Northeastern Illinois University and the National University of Health Sciences. His certifications include Certified Chiropractic Extremity Practitioner, Diplomat of the American Academy of Pain Practitioneres, Impairment Rating Certification, Level 1 Accreditation for Colorado Division of Worker's Compensation, Certified Colorado High School Athletic Association Chiropractic Provider, Certified in Zone Nutrition Program, and a graduate of the Institute for Functional Medicine. He is the company chiropractor for the Colorado Ballet Company.

Besides being an accomplished practitioner, Dr. Troeger is an esteemed lecturer--giving talks on Soft Tissue Injury and Treatment, and Soft Tissue Techniques--and is a member of numerous associations including the Colorado Chiropractic Society where he served as a board member as well as vice president and president; the Colorado Chiropractic Society where he held many offices including chairman of the board and president; the American Academy of Chiropractic Physicians, American Chiropractic Association, the A.C.A. Council on Nutrition, the A.C.A. Council on Diagnostic Imaging, and the A.C.A. Council on Sports Injuries and Physical Fitness. Dr. Troeger is also a member of the Foundation of Chiropractic Education and Research, the Christian Chiropractic Association and a member of Sigma Phi Kappa Fraternity.

He has produced and written professional training videos (Dynamic Stretch and Strength Training) and won numerous awards including the Outstanding Young Chiropractor of the Year in 1982, Outstanding Young Men of America in 1983, Excellence in Patient Education and Communication Award in 2006, Chiropractic Distinguished Quality Service Honor Five Star Award, Integrity and Management in 2007, the International Who's Who of Entrepreneurs Award in 2001--among others.   His practice is located in Denver, Colorado.

Deborah has a Bachelor's of Science degree in Financial Management from Southwest Missouri State University. She worked in the telecommunications industry for twelve years. Her job experience ranged from customer service, system design and project management to sales. In 1997 Deborah went back to school to earn her Masters Degree in Counseling from Colorado Christian University. She graduated in 2000 and began private practice, specializing in sexual abuse, dealing with issues regarding: self image, confidence, anger, boundaries, and emotional eating. She became a Certified Clinical Hypnotherapist in 2004 and began focusing on weight loss, combining counseling with her skills as a hypnotherapist to help improve people's health and mental and spiritual well being.

Born and raised in Missouri. Deborah moved to Denver, CO in 1991 with her 2 children. She is married to Dr. Steven Troeger, DC and has two step children and three grand children. In her spare time she enjoys, snow skiing, water skiing, bare foot water skiing and running.

Chapter Eighteen: High Tech Solution To Weight Loss
by Patrick K. Porter, Ph.D.

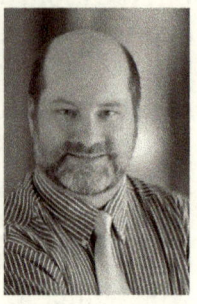

Patrick K. Porter, Ph.D. is an award-winning author, entrepreneur, and experienced speaker. With 24 years of experience operating the largest self-help franchise, he has become a highly sought-after expert within the personal improvement industry. He is the Creator of the ZenFrames, Behavioral Repatterning Device (BRD) which is uses by the HealthSource Doctors to help people overcome stress and insomnia, lose weight, stop smoking, manage pain, accelerate learning, and much more.

He is the author of the bestselling book, *Awaken the Genius, Mind Technology for the 21st Century*, which was awarded "Best How-To Book of 1994" by the North American Book Dealers Exchange.

He is also author of *Discover the Language of the Mind*, and *Six Secrets of G.E.N.I.U.S.* Dr. Porter has produced an arsenal of more than 300 audio-recorded motivational programs and creative visualization processes, and has sold more than three million books and recordings worldwide. The material from this chapter has been adapted from his book, Thrive In Overdrive, "How to Navigate Your Overloaded Lifestyle."

Chapter Nineteen: Recognize Hidden Thyroid Problems In Weight Loss
by Mark Lewis, DC

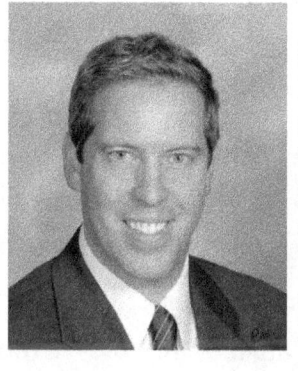

Dr. Lewis graduated with his master's degree from George Mason University in 1995 and subsequently graduated from Texas Chiropractic College in 2005. He is a member of the American Chiropractic Association, the Florida Chiropractic Association and the Council on Diagnosis and Internal Disorders. He is a member of the Omega Psi Honor society and was the Student American Chiropractic Society Representative from 2002 through 2005.

His post graduate training includes many hours covering Internal Medicine and Clinical Nutrition, Chiropractic Family Practice, Functional Medicine, DOT Physical exam, Acupuncture and numerous other subjects. He is the author of several articles in publication including, "Living Out East", "Florida Women Today", and "Positive Change."

Dr. Lewis has given hundreds of presentations and health screenings including speaking to elementary schools, school districts, banks and community organizations. His speaking engagements have included Health and Wellness; Back Pain; Arthritis Fibromyalgia and Chronic Fatigue; Thyroid Dysfunction; Digestive Disorders, Food Allergies and Celiac Disease.

Dr. Lewis believes in a detailed diagnostic approach to identify the source of pain and body dysfunction. He incorporates chiropractic, manual therapy, therapeutic exercise and the effective application of nutritional products in his comprehensive treatment plans. His practice, Essential Wellness, PLLC, is in Bradenton, Florida.

Chapter Twenty: The Importance of Water
by Jon Steffins, DC

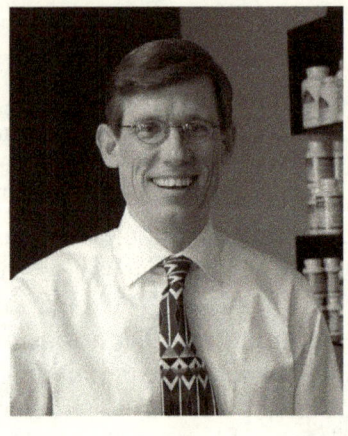

Dr. Steffins received his undergraduate training from Harding University and his chiropractic training from Parker College of Chiropractic where he served as Student Senate Treasurer and Masters Circle Club President and graduated with Clinic Honors. His post graduate training includes training in the pain neutralization technique, clinical nutrition for pain, inflammation and tissue healing, Board certified physiotherapy, and community based wellness partnership.

He is a member of the Unified Chiropractic Association of Oklahoma, the Oklahoma Chiropractic Independent Physicians Association, American Chiropractic Association, Christian Chiropractic Association, and a board member of the Optimists Club.

Dr. Steffins' Health Source Chiropractic clinic is located in Tulsa Oklahoma where he provides chiropractic and progressive rehabilitation care.

Chapter Twenty One: Exercise and Weight Loss

by Jeff Wisdo, DC

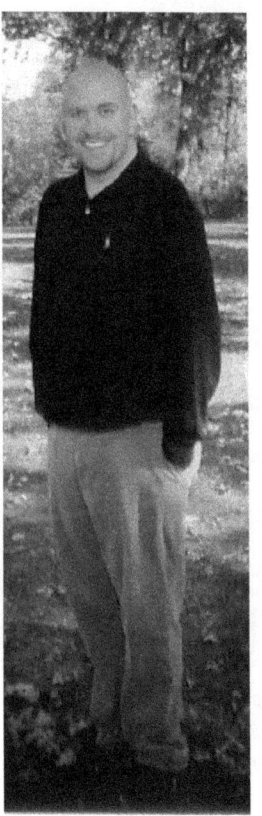

Dr. Jeff Wisdo graduated from Palmer College of Chiropractic in Davenport, Iowa in 1999. He joined HealthSource first as a franchisee then later that same year became the Regional Developer for Minnesota. Currently with his two partners, he is helping other chiropractors change their chiropractic practices into strong, stable and successful businesses.

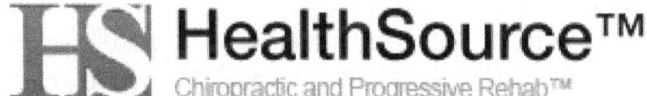

Franchise Opportunities

Hire A Consultant Because Your Practice Is Shrinking? Tried That Already? Get more information at: http://franchisees.healthsourcechiro.com.

HEALTHSOURCE ECLUSIVE WEIGHT-LOSS CREATIVE VISUALIZATION & RELAXATION SYSTEM

HealthSource is proud to announce its partnership with America's top expert in mind-based weight-loss, Patrick K. Porter, Ph.D.

Dr. Porter has designed an exclusive mental coaching program just for you, the HealthSource patient, that will not only kick-start your weight-loss program but also give you the proper mindset for keeping off your weight for the rest of your life.

Dr. Porter uses Creative Visualization & Relaxation (Behavioral Repatterning) sessions to accelerate the already astounding results patients are getting with the HealthSource **Six Keys to Success** treatment for obesity and excessive weight. Each week, you will focus on one or more of the **Six Keys to Success** by relaxing daily with your Behavioral Re-patterning Device (BRD) guided by Dr. Porter as your personal coach.

By the time you have completed the HealthSource *Six Keys to Success weight-loss plan*, combined with Dr. Porter's mental coaching system, you will be too smart and too health savvy to ever go back to the habits that caused you to gain weight in the past. Our goal is your goal—for you to take your weight off and never have to diet again!

HSWC01 – Breaking the Chains of Weight-Loss Resistance Syndrome

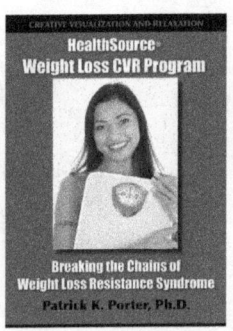

Dr. Porter has put together this session to help you change the mental patterns that run through your mind each time you make a food choice. You will create healthy behaviors to replace the unwanted overweight habits that in the past sabotaged your success. Why hold on to the detrimental thought patterns that threaten your health and keep you from achieving permanent weight-loss success? Now you can simply sit back, relax, and change the way you think about yourself and food. By establishing the correct relationship between you and food, you will eliminate the habit of weight-loss failure for good.

HSWC02 – Creating A Diet That Works For You

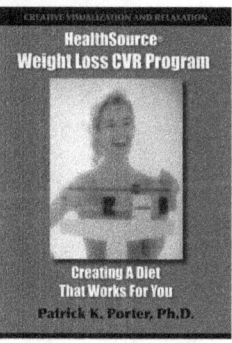

During this session, you will begin by becoming honest with yourself about how much you eat, how frequently you eat, and the number of calories of fat, protein, and carbohydrates you consume. With this knowledge working at the other-than-conscious level of your mind, you will easily cut out snacks and eat smaller portions. Dr. Patrick Porter will have you looking forward to eating the right foods that will stimulate your body to transform into a fat burning machine.

HSWC03 - Supercharge Your Joy For Exercise

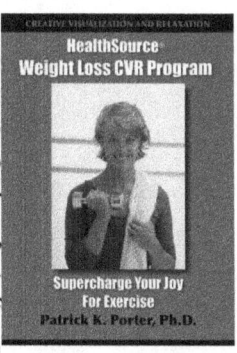

As you go through HealthSource's proven weight-loss system, the goal is to establish habits that will keep you at your ideal weight forever. With this in mind, Dr. Porter has designed this mental exercise program that will put the joy of movement back into your life. Through the power of your own mind, you will discover ways to enjoy exercise and to make it a fundamental part of the healthy new you. When you build these habits with the help of your mind, you will be making positive changes to ensure an excellent quality of life at every age.

HSWC04 – Turn Your Body Into A Fat Burning Machine

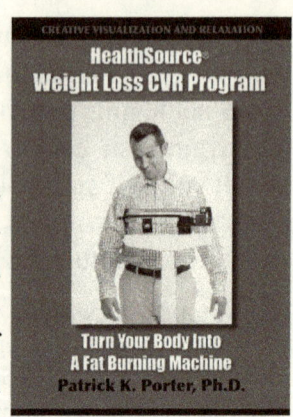

You are the sum total of the foods that you consume, the beverages you drink, and the attitude you keep in consciousness. Stimulating your metabolism and taking off weight cannot occur in a dehydrated state. In this visualization, you will experience Dr. Porter's proven technique to get you drinking and savoring water on a daily basis. You will learn to balance your life while building subconscious triggers that will have you drinking 6-8 glasses of water a day without any effort on your part. This will stimulate fat burning throughout your day and even at the deepest level of sleep.

HSWC05 – Living Your Life As A Naturally Thin Person

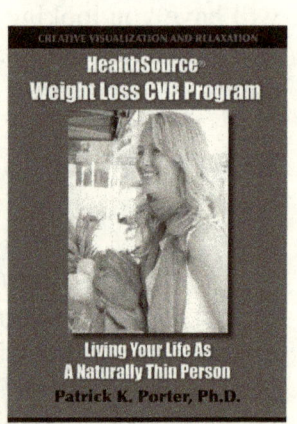

Most people are unaware that they regularly eat when they are not truly hungry. In fact, one study showed that 80% of the time when we put food into our mouths, we are not physiologically hungry. With this visualization, you will mentally rehearse the behaviors of a naturally thin person. Get ready to eliminate the habits of eating due to stress, boredom, anger, or fatigue. No longer will negative emotions control you. Even with external cues like the smell or sight of food or the appetite triggers of social situations, you will feel empowered knowing that nothing tastes as good as thin and healthy feels.

HSW06 – Eliminate Overweight Behaviors

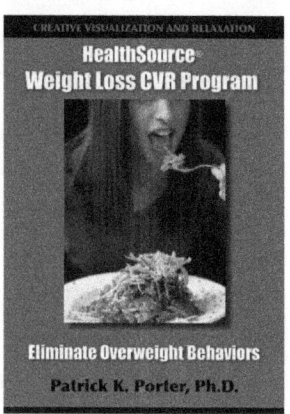

Those who have dieted regularly know that behaviors are the most challenging factor in weight-loss. Yet to make a permanent positive change in your health, developing appropriate eating behavior is a must. At HealthSource we know that returning to your natural weight is just one of the steps you are taking to safeguard your health. That's why Dr. Porter has designed this program with a lifestyle change in mind. With the old behaviors gone, you will always feel empowered to think before you eat!

HSWC07 – Erase Triggers That Caused The Weight In The First Place

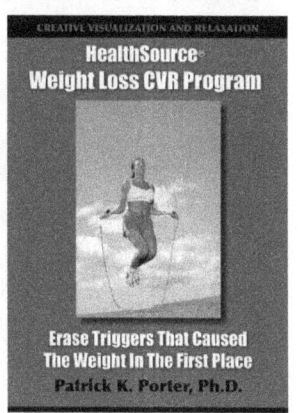

Many people unwittingly use food like a drug—for stress relief, comfort, or escape. With this breakthrough process, Dr. Porter will help you interrupt or eliminate these old triggers and free you from any guilt or shame associated with past patterns. You will use the power of possibility thinking instead of food when outside stimuli would otherwise prompt you to consume fattening foods. You will rehearse positive behaviors that energize and refresh your mind and body.

HSWC08 - Developing the "HealthSource" Mind Set for Life!

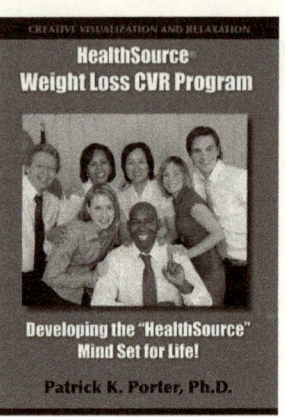

Your mental outlook is key to success in anything you do in life. As Henry Ford said, "If you think you can, or if you think you can't, you are right." During this visualization, you will preview your success in the weight-loss process, all the while gaining positive life skills. You will learn why health is wealth and how the HealthSource system is designed to get you from where you are now to living out a day-to-day plan for success.

HSWC09 – Planning Your Life Naturally Thin

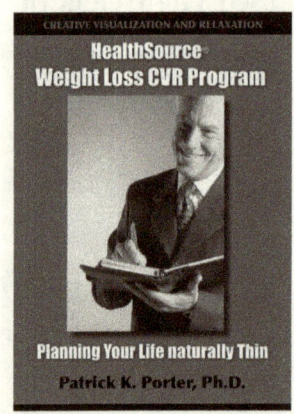

During this session, Dr. Porter will guide you to forget about past dieting experiences that didn't work, and focus on the HealthSource System that does work. While relaxing to soothing music and Dr. Porter's encouraging words, you will imagine daily success. As you steadily return to your natural weight, you will notice small changes taking place in your body. Dr. Porter encourages you to celebrate these "little victories," giving you the momentum to make better choices, see faster results, and propel you toward the ideal weight you have set for yourself.

HSWC10 – The Plan Works... So Work the Plan!

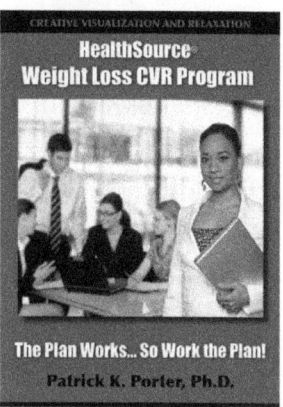

Most people are seeking a magic pill for weight-loss, but you'll be ahead of that game, because you'll be using the magic of your own mind! With this session, you will put your expectations in perspective so you can apply the core steps of the HealthSource system on a daily basis. The result? Lasting change without the negative side-effects associated with medication. You will learn how to use the world's most powerful pharmacy . . . your human brain. Once you learn these steps, your success will be on autopilot!

HSWC11 Making the Lasting Connection

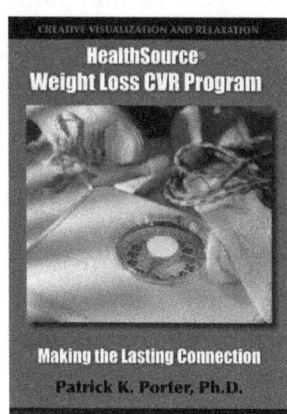

The key to maintaining your natural weight is to "love thyself." With this session, you will decide to take off your excess weight not so you can become an extraordinary person, but because you are one. This single shift in your consciousness will improve your attitude and health by leaps and bounds. Once the full resources of your mind are working for you, what can possibly be against you? Now is the time to eliminate once and for all the self-sabotaging habits that used to prevent you from achieving lasting happiness.

HSWC12 – Unlock Your Creative Genius

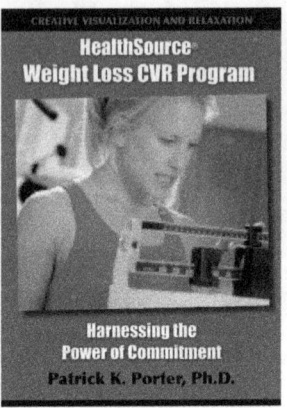

Those who win in life are those who make their own rules. In this relaxation, Dr. Porter helps you develop a personalized system for eating healthy and living life to its fullest. No one knows your strengths and weaknesses better than you do. You will use your creativity to find the parts of your program that you'll find easier as well as those that you'll find more challenging and then plan for every contingency so you will succeed effortlessly.

HSWC13 – Harnessing the Power of Commitment

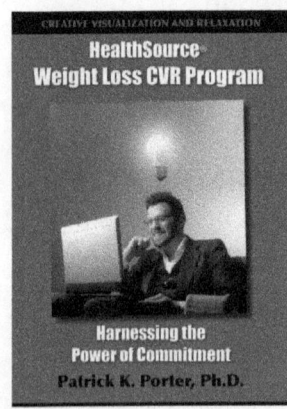

Throughout your mental training, you have been learning to use the most powerful force in the universe—the power of thought. Now, by using your mental powerhouse, you will no longer give in to temptation. Rather, you will embrace the expression, "There is no failure, only feedback." You will commit to making the lifelong changes in behavior and lifestyle that bring about lasting weight-loss—and you will vow to never diet again!

"What the mind can conceive and believe, it will achieve!"

Transform Your iPod or any MP3 Player into a Behavioral Repatterning Device (BRD)

Find Out What You Can Achieve When You Dare to Relax!

BRD + Your Brain = Success!

ZenFrames are an extraordinary new technology that delivers gentle pulses of light and sound and combines it with guided visualization and soothing music to take you to the profound levels of relaxation known for focus, learning, achievement, and healing.

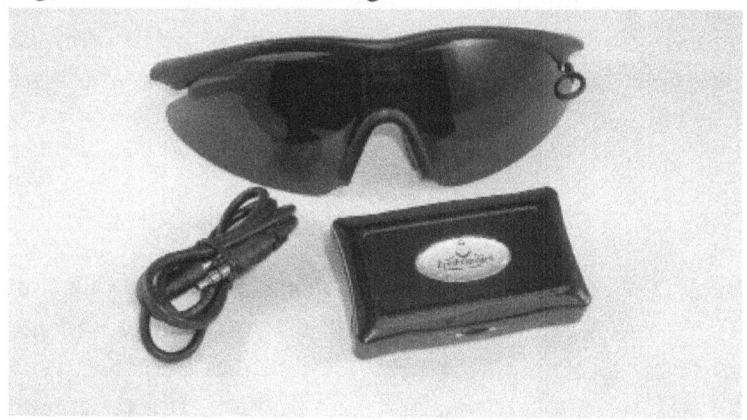

Want to lose weight? Just click on one of the titles, then relax and let your mind do the rest.

Is playing better golf your thing? Any of more than a dozen visualization sessions can easily help you master the game.

Maybe you just want a little time to get away from life's stresses. No problem. Simply choose a program from the stress-free series and enjoy a mental vacation.

With hundreds of programs to choose from at ZenFramesBRD.com, there's simply no limit to how good you can feel and what you can achieve.

If you want to get more done in less time then the BRD is for you!

Your BRD comes with everything you need—you simply plug your BRD into the earphone jack of your iPod or MP3 player and you're ready to dream big! Plus, when you register your BRD, you get your own personal webpage for downloading new processes, tracking your progress and receiving updates. There's no software to install. You can take your Behavioral Repatterning Device with you wherever you go!

Four Mind Technologies in One Mind-Blowing Pair of Glasses!

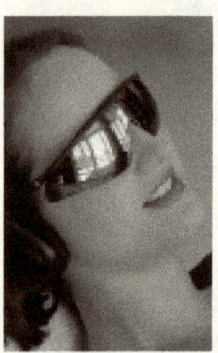

Light Frequencies Distinctive flashing light patterns train your brain to operate in the best possible mode for creativity, focus, and mindfulness. If you are the type who likes to get things done, this form of brainwave entrainment can transform you into a mental powerhouse with the right mindset, energy and clarity to accomplish just about anything.

Binaural Beats Put simply, these are imbedded tones that the brain naturally follows into states of deep relaxation. Within minutes your brain reaches extraordinary levels of performance that would otherwise take years of practice to achieve.

Creative Visualization/Relaxation (Behavioral Repatterning) CVR can help you change the way you view yourself and your life. Once you have a new image of yourself—as a healthy, happy, optimistic person—your fears and frustrations fade away and you no longer let small things stress you. Behavioral repatterning makes sure you are focusing on everything you want out of life so you can have it, effortlessly!

Mind-Music The music you hear on every PorterVision process is designed to create a full 360 degree experience that floods your mind with beautiful images and peaceful thoughts.

Dare to Relax with behavioral repatterning and You'll Enjoy all these Benefits and More!

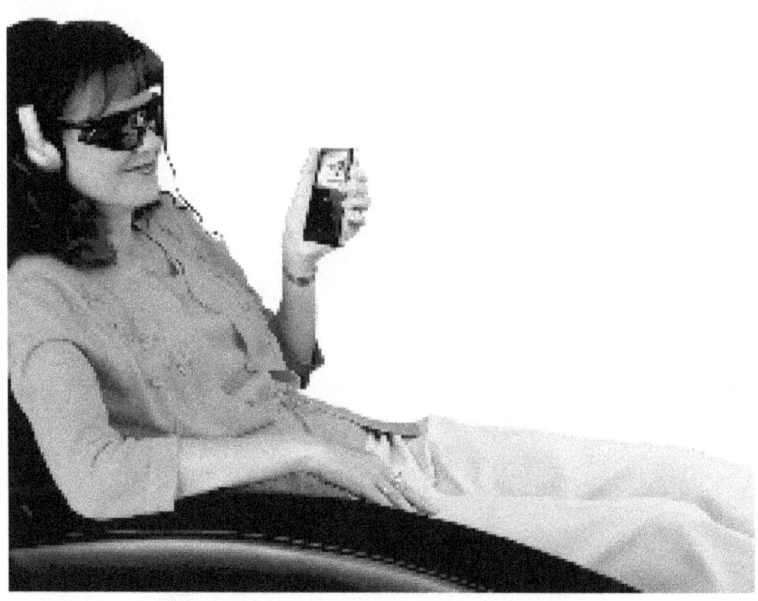

For more information go to: www.healthsourcechiro.com